Clinical Skills
for Pharmacists
A Patient-Focused Approach

Clinical Skills for Pharmacists
A Patient-Focused Approach

Second Edition

Karen J. Tietze, PharmD

Professor of Clinical Pharmacy
Philadelphia College of Pharmacy and Science
University of the Sciences in Philadelphia
Philadelphia, Pennsylvania

with 45 illustrations

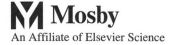
An Affiliate of Elsevier Science

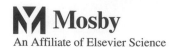

Mosby

An Affiliate of Elsevier Science

11830 Westline Industrial Drive
St. Louis, Missouri 63146

Notice

Pharmacology is an ever-changing field. Standard safety precautions must be followed, but as new research and clinical experience broaden our knowledge, changes in treatment and drug therapy may become necessary or appropriate. Readers are advised to check the most current product information provided by the manufacturer of each drug to be administered to verify the recommended dose, the method and duration of administration, and con-traindications. It is the responsibility of the licensed prescriber, relying on experience and knowledge of the patient, to determine dosages and the best treatment for each individual patient. Neither the publisher nor the author assumes any liability for any injury and/or damage to persons or property arising from this publication.

The Publisher

Previous editions copyrighted 1997

Library of Congress Cataloging-in-Publication Data

Tietze, Karen J.
    Clinical skills for pharmacists : a patient-focused approach / Karen J. Tietze—2nd ed.
        p. cm.
    Includes bibliographical references and index.
    ISBN 0-323-02473-4
        1. Pharmacy. 2. Pharmacy—Practice. 3. Communication in pharmacy. I. Title.
    RS91.T54 2003
    615'.1—dc21

                                                                        2003059986

Publishing Director: Linda Duncan
Acquisitions Editor: Kellie White
Developmental Editor: Kim Fons
Publishing Services Manager: John Rogers
Design Manager: Bill Drone

Printed in the United States of America

Last digit is the print number: 9   8   7   6   5   4   3   2   1

To my students.

Preface

In the preface to the first edition of *Clinical Skills for Pharmacists* I described how the book was developed, the organizational structure and format of the book, and my hopes for the book. I ended the preface by stating that the book was a work in progress and that all suggestions for improvement were welcome. Although I thought the book was unique and hoped it would find a useful niche within the profession, I was unsure how it would be accepted. I have been quite surprised by the overwhelming positive response the book has elicited. Although my students delight in pointing out the occasional typographical error or inconsistency, feedback regarding the style and content has been consistently positive. The book seems to have found a niche as a unique compilation of skill-related topics, complementary to clerkship manuals and physical assessment and ethics textbooks.

The organizational structure of this second edition is unchanged from that of the first edition. Each chapter begins with specific learning objectives and ends with 10 self-assessment questions. Chapters discussing fundamental skills (communication skills, physical assessment skills, and laboratory and diagnostic information) precede chapters on more specific and applied skills (the patient case presentation, therapeutic planning, and monitoring). Each chapter builds on and is integrated with prior chapters.

The second edition has been completely revised and updated. Several new figures have been added. Information regarding new opportunities in board certification and certificate programs has been added to Chapter 1. Chapter 3, Taking Medication Histories, has been revised to include more information about alternative remedies. The medication history checklist has been revised to include alternative remedies. The inconsistencies in the medication history documentation examples have been corrected. Chapter 4, Physical Assessment Skills, has been reorganized to follow a more obvious organ system–specific IPPA (inspection, percussion, palpation, and auscultation) sequence. All Système Internationale units have been deleted throughout the text. Discussions of several new labs have been added to Chapter 5, Review of Laboratory and Diagnostic Tests. The patient case example in Chapter 6, The Patient Case Presentation, has been simplified. Chapter 8, Monitoring Drug Therapies, and Chapter 9, Researching and Providing Drug Information, have been updated to reflect advances in electronic access to information. Chapter 10, Ethics in Pharmacy and Health Care, has been updated to reflect the most current professional codes.

This book remains a work in progress. Comments and suggestions for improvement are always welcomed.

Karen J. Tietze

Acknowledgments

It is impossible to individually thank all those who contributed to the development of this book. I hope that my global thanks reach all the individuals who have contributed to the development and content of this book. I thank all my students who continue to teach me how to learn clinical pharmacy skills. I also thank my colleagues at the University of the Sciences in Philadelphia whose moral support during the developmental stages of the book and the writing of the second edition was invaluable.

Special thanks to the following individuals who provided detailed reviews of one or more chapters when the book was being developed: Jerry L. Bauman, Pharm.D.; Janice A. Gaska, Pharm.D.; Arthur I. Jacknowitz, Pharm.D.; Paul L. Ranelli, Ph.D.; and Timothy H. Self, Pharm.D.

I am especially indebted to Dr. Janice Gaska. Our original plan was to coauthor the book. We spent countless hours planning the book before she changed careers. The book reflects both of our philosophies and is much better than I could have created on my own.

No book can succeed without the resources and support of the publisher. I have been incredibly lucky to work with very talented editors from Mosby, Inc., an affiliate of Elsevier Science (USA). My editorial team for the first edition included Sandra Parker, Developmental Editor; Laura MacAdam, Developmental Editor; Jennifer Roche, Acquisitions Editor; and Jennifer Furey, Production Editor. Their guidance and enthusiasm were invaluable. The editors for the second edition, Kellie White, Editor, and Kim Fons, Senior Developmental Editor, continue that tradition. Their "can do" attitude and never-failing enthusiasm for the book kept me motivated and on track with our very ambitious production timeline.

Finally, thanks to my family for their support and understanding of what it takes to get this type of project completed.

Karen J. Tietze

Contents

Introduction: The Practice of Clinical Pharmacy

CHAPTER 1

Learning Objectives

- Define *pharmaceutical care* and identify the four outcomes that improve a patient's quality of life.
- List the knowledge and skills needed for patient-focused pharmacy practice.
- State the eligibility requirements for board certification and identify the areas for which board certification is available.
- Differentiate between residencies and fellowships in terms of definition, length of training, and mechanisms for credentialing.
- Differentiate between board certification, added qualifications, and certificate programs in terms of eligibility and requirements.
- Identify and differentiate among the various types of health care settings and environments.
- State the purpose of the medical team and identify the roles and responsibilities of each team member.
- Identify and describe unresolved health care system issues.

*P*harmacy practice is moving toward a model that integrates patient-focused care (also known as *patient-centered care*) and drug distribution services. To be successful, pharmacists must understand and speak the language of the health care system and function in a system that to the uninitiated is foreign and excessively complex. The variety of providers, rapidly evolving types of health care delivery systems, and complexities of relationships among the various health care professionals working within the health care system add to the confusion. This chapter describes patient-focused pharmacy practice and the clinical environment in which patient-focused pharmacists function.

PATIENT-FOCUSED PHARMACY PRACTICE

The term *clinical pharmacy* historically described patient-oriented rather than product-oriented pharmacy practice. The term *clinical pharmacist* was used to describe a pharmacist whose primary job was to interact with the health care team, interview and assess patients, make patient-specific therapeutic recommendations, monitor patient response to drug therapy, and provide drug information. Clinical pharmacists, working primarily in acute care settings, were viewed as "drug experts"; other pharmacists could occasionally use "clinical" skills, but they remained focused on product management. The profession of pharmacy has evolved to the point that many pharmacists find the term *clinical pharmacy* redundant; the term *pharmacist* implies the integration of patient- and product-oriented pharmacy practice.

The term *pharmaceutical care* is used to describe the broad-based, patient-focused responsibilities of pharmacists. Hepler and Strand define pharmaceutical care as the "responsible provision of drug therapy for the purpose of achieving definite outcomes that improve a patient's quality of life."[1] The four outcomes identified include the following:

1. Cure of disease
2. Elimination or reduction of symptoms
3. Arrest or slowing of a disease process
4. Prevention of disease or symptoms

Pharmaceutical care requires an expert knowledge of therapeutics; a good understanding of disease processes; knowledge of drug products; strong communication skills; drug monitoring, drug information, and therapeutic planning skills; and the ability to assess and interpret physical assessment findings (Figure 1-1).

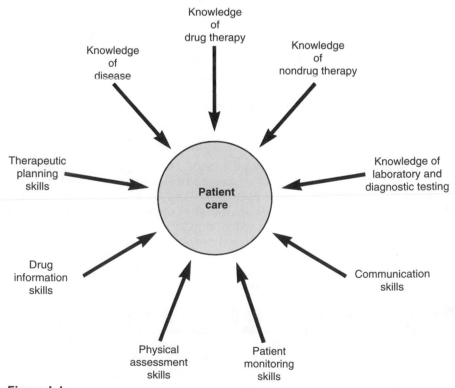

Figure 1-1
Patient Care.
Patient care requires integration of knowledge and skills.

SITES AND TYPES OF PRACTICE

Patient-focused pharmacy practice is performed everywhere patients interact with the health care system, including teaching and community hospitals, outpatient clinics, community pharmacies, long-term care facilities, and home health care. Pharmacists, like other health care professionals, specialize in specialty practice areas such as pediatrics, critical care, nutrition, and cardiology. Some specialty practice areas (e.g., infectious disease, nutrition) parallel and are similar to traditional medical specialty or subspecialty areas. Other specialty practice areas (e.g., drug information, pharmacokinetics) are unique to pharmacy (Box 1-1).

Patient-focused pharmacists work closely with physicians and other health care professionals to provide optimal patient care. Some pharmacists in traditional product-centered practice settings use clinical pharmacy skills in a limited capacity, such as when they obtain a medication history or triage a patient to self-care with nonprescription drugs. Some pharmacists have no traditional product-centered responsibilities and instead provide full-time pharmaceutical care. Regardless of the setting and the degree to which patient-focused skills are used, pharmaceutical care is an integral part of the practice of pharmacy.

The only requirements for providing patient-focused services are adequate background and training. Pharmacists with Bachelor of Science in Pharmacy degrees or Doctor of Pharmacy degrees provide patient-focused services. The largest difference between the two educational programs is that Doctor of Pharmacy programs provide more intensive experience and training in the data and skills necessary for patient-focused practice than traditional 5-year baccalaureate programs. Postgraduate training programs provide the pharmacist with even more intensive supervised experience and training.

CERTIFICATION AND ADDED QUALIFICATIONS

Board certification (official recognition of specific knowledge and skills) is achieved in addition to state and federal professional licensure. Some employers require board certification for specific jobs, such as nutrition support and clinical coordinator positions; other employers reward pharmacists who become board certified with additional career advancement opportunities and salary differentials. The Board of Pharmaceutical Specialties (BPS), created in 1976 by the American Pharmaceutical

---

BOX 1-1

Patient-Focused Practice Areas

Ambulatory care	Nephrology
Critical care	Obstetrics and gynecology
Drug information	Pulmonary disease
Geriatrics and long-term care	Psychiatry
Internal medicine and subspecialties	Rheumatology
Cardiology	Nuclear pharmacy
Endocrinology	Nutrition
Gastroenterology	Pediatrics
Infectious disease	Pharmacokinetics
Neurology	Surgery

Association, is responsible for setting standards for certification and recertification and for administering the certification and recertification processes. Board certification by written examination is available in Nuclear Pharmacy, Nutrition Support Pharmacy, Oncology Pharmacy, Pharmacotherapy, and Psychiatric Pharmacy; certification of other areas is under consideration. Pharmacists with advanced education (Doctor of Pharmacy degrees) and training or equivalent experience are eligible for certification. The BPS requires that board-certified pharmacists complete periodic recredentialing requirements, typically specified types of continuing education or reexamination. Board certified pharmacists are entitled to denote the accomplishment in their title (Board Certified Nuclear Pharmacist [BCNP], Board Certified Nutrition Support Pharmacist [BCNSP], Board Certified Oncology Pharmacist [BCOP], Board Certified Pharmacotherapy Specialist [BCPS], and Board Certified Psychiatric Pharmacist [BCPP]).

Board Certified Pharmacotherapy Specialists are eligible for Added Qualifications in cardiology and infectious diseases. Administered by the BPS, Added Qualifications recognize a high level of training and experience within a BPS-recognized specialty practice area. Candidates for Added Qualifications are judged on the contents of a portfolio documenting the candidates advanced training and experience. Individuals who have achieved Added Qualification status are reassessed every 7 years.

POSTGRADUATE TRAINING

Pharmacy graduates obtain additional experience, knowledge, and skills by completing a variety of residency and fellowship postgraduate training and certificate programs. Most residency and fellowship programs require candidates to have either entry-level or postbaccalaureate Doctor of Pharmacy degrees. The American Society of Health-System Pharmacists (ASHP) publishes a directory of ASHP-accredited residency programs. The American College of Clinical Pharmacy (ACCP) publishes a directory of residency and fellowship programs offered by members of the ACCP. Both directories are updated annually.

A *residency* is an "organized, directed, postgraduate training program in a defined area of pharmacy practice."[2] The ASHP accredits residency programs. Residencies provide pharmacists 1 to 2 years of supervised experience in practice and management activities. Residencies may be general, providing broad-based experiences, or specialized in focused areas such as ambulatory care, drug information, and pediatrics (Box 1-2). Residents generally gain experience by providing a variety of inpatient and outpatient pharmacy services. Most residencies are based in hospitals;

BOX 1-2

Postgraduate Pharmacy Residency Programs

Administration	Family medicine	Nutrition
Ambulatory care	Gastroenterology	Oncology
Cardiology	General medicine	Pediatrics
Community pharmacy	Geriatrics	Pharmacokinetics
Critical care	Hospital pharmacy	Pharmacotherapy
Dermatology	Infectious disease	Psychiatry
Drug information	Nephrology	Toxicology

however, increased interest in community pharmacy and ambulatory care residencies has resulted in the creation of an increasing number of community pharmacy and ambulatory care residency programs.

A *fellowship* is a highly individualized program designed to prepare the pharmacist to become an independent researcher.[2] Currently no mechanism for accreditation of fellowship programs is available. However, the ACCP Fellowship Review Committee conducts a voluntary peer-review program. As of 2002, 16 fellowship programs were recognized as meeting ACCP fellowship program guidelines. Fellowship applicants are expected to have completed Doctor of Pharmacy and residency programs or to have equivalent experience. Fellowships provide pharmacists with 1 to 3 years of supervised research experience in highly focused areas such as pharmacokinetics, oncology, and nephrology (Box 1-3). Fellows spend approximately 80% of their time in research-related activities.

Certificate programs are topic-specific educational programs open to all pharmacists. A certificate is awarded after successful completion of the disease-specific educational program and examination. The National Institute for Standards in Pharmacist Credentialing (NISPC), formed in 1998 by the American Pharmaceutical Association, the National Association of Boards of Pharmacy, the National Association of Chain Drug Stores, and the National Community Pharmacists Association, administers a nationally recognized credentialing process that results in a Certified Disease Manager (CDM) designation in anticoagulation, asthma, diabetes, or dyslipidemia for pharmacists who successfully pass a written examination. Non-NISPC certificate programs, ranging from short, weekend educational programs to multiple hours of coursework, are available. The National Certification Board for Diabetes Educators (NCBDE), an independent organization, grants certification (Certified Diabetes Educator; CDE) to qualified health care professionals.

THE CLINICAL ENVIRONMENT

Health care is provided in many different settings (Box 1-4). Examples of outpatient (ambulatory) settings include private offices, outpatient clinics, day surgery units (also known as *short procedure units*), and emergency rooms. Acute care hospitals provide inpatient care. Patients are hospitalized for major surgery, treatment of acute disorders, and diagnostic evaluations and procedures. Long-term care facilities, such as nursing homes and rehabilitation centers, provide health care for patients who

---

BOX 1-3

Postgraduate Pharmacy Fellowship Training Programs

Ambulatory care	Family medicine	Oncology
Analgesia	Gastroenterology	Pediatrics
Cardiology	General medicine	Pharmacodynamics
Critical care	Geriatrics	Pharmacokinetics
Dermatology	Infectious disease	Psychiatry
Drug development	Nephrology	Pulmonary disease
Drug information	Neurology	Rheumatology
Drug metabolism	Nutrition	

BOX 1-4

Health Care Settings

OUTPATIENT	INPATIENT
Clinics	Hospitals
Day surgery units	**LONG-TERM CARE FACILITIES**
Emergency rooms	Rehabilitation centers
Home health care	Skilled nursing homes
Private offices	

require skilled management of chronic disorders. Home health care services are available for chronically ill and disabled patients.

Physicians provide inpatient and outpatient health care services in individual and group practices. Group practices consist of physicians with the same type of medical practice (e.g., family medicine) or physicians with different specialties (e.g., internal medicine, family medicine, and obstetrics and gynecology). Physician practices changed dramatically in response to the 1990's evolution of health care delivery from traditional fee-for-service (FFS) indemnity insurance plans in which patients were free to select any physician they wanted to managed care insurance plans in which patients were restricted in their choices. Many different alliances have formed among physicians, health care institutions, and insurers, including physician networks, prepaid group practices, and integrated delivery systems.

Clinics, often affiliated with major medical centers and hospitals, are located in a variety of outpatient settings, including community centers, medical offices, and freestanding clinics. Clinics serve general unrestricted patient populations or very specific patient populations. Clinics serving a specific patient population usually are named after that population (e.g., hypertension clinic, diabetes clinic, anticoagulation clinic, medication refill clinic). Several clinics may share the same physical space; in this situation the schedule is set to allow each clinic to have a unique weekly or daily schedule (e.g., anticoagulation clinic on Tuesday afternoons, diabetes clinic on Wednesday mornings, hypertension clinic on Friday mornings).

Hospitals are identified as public, private, or federal hospitals, depending on the funding source. Public hospitals are publicly funded and provide health care services to all patients, regardless of the patient's type of insurance or ability to pay for the health care services. Some cities and states pay for public hospital services from tax revenues. Private hospitals are privately funded institutions whose services are generally not available, except for emergency care, to patients who are not part of the private group. The federal government funds federal hospitals. The Veterans Administration hospital system is an extensive nationwide system of hospitals, clinics, and nursing homes funded by the federal government to provide health care services to American armed forces veterans.

Hospitals, regardless of the funding source, may be affiliated with medical schools. These hospitals, known as *teaching hospitals,* provide training sites for physicians and other health care professionals. Community-based, nonteaching hospitals are sometimes called *community hospitals.* Some hospitals, recognized for their highly specialized services (e.g., pediatrics, oncology, cardiology) and large referral patient population, are known as *tertiary hospitals.*

HEALTH CARE PROFESSIONALS

Health care professionals include physicians, pharmacists, and nurses. Allied health care professionals, also known as *paramedicals,* provide health care services and perform tasks under the direction of physicians (Box 1-5).

Physicians. Physicians, doctors who have medical or osteopathic degrees, are generally considered the health care team leader and have ultimate legal responsibility for the patient. Allopathic physicians rely on standard treatment modalities; osteopathic physicians use the additional technique of spine and joint manipulation to treat disease.

Physicians practice medicine in many general and specialty areas (Box 1-6). Family practice physicians, general internal medicine physicians, and pediatric physicians treat patients with a variety of diseases. Specialists such as nephrologists and cardiologists treat patients within a narrow spectrum of disease. Many internists (physicians specializing in internal medicine) elect to specialize in a subspecialty such a nephrology, cardiology, oncology, pulmonary disease, infectious disease, or neurology. Some confusion regarding certification and specialization may occur because physicians do not have to be certified to practice specialty or subspecialty areas.

Physicians are licensed by individual states and credentialed by national examination. A physician must graduate from an accredited medical school, receive passing grades on the medical licensure examination (usually the National Board of Medical Examiners examination), and (in most states) complete 1 year of an accredited residency program to become licensed to practice medicine. Relicensure requires successful completion of specified continuing medical education programs. Most physicians obtain 1 year or more of supervised experience in residency programs; some complete additional training in highly specialized fellowship programs. The length of the residency program depends on the specialty or subspecialty. Internal medicine residencies are typically 3 years in duration; surgical residencies may be 5 to 7 years.

Nurses. Nurses care for the physical and psychosocial needs of patients and carry out physician-directed orders regarding patient care. Nurses perform many routine

---

BOX 1-5

Allied Health Care Professionals

Anesthesiologist's assistant	Medical technologist
Cardiovascular technologist	Occupational therapist
Cytotechnologist	Ophthalmic medical assistant
Diagnostic medical sonographer	Perfusionist
Electroencephalographic technologist	Physician assistant
Emergency medical technician	Radiation therapy technologist
Histologic technician	Radiographer
Medical assistant	Respiratory therapist
Medical illustrator	Respiratory therapy technician
Medical laboratory technician	Specialist in blood bank technology
Medical record administrator	Surgeon's assistant/technologist
Medical record technician	

BOX 1-6

Physician Practice Areas

MEDICAL	**SURGICAL**
Allergy and immunology	Cardiothoracic
Dermatology	Colorectal
Family practice	General
General practice	Neurologic
Internal medicine	Obstetric and gynecologic
Cardiovascular medicine	Ophthalmologic
Critical care	Orthopedic
Endocrinology	Otorhinolaryngologic
Gastroenterology	Plastic
Hematology	Urologic
Infectious disease	**OTHERS**
Medical oncology	Anesthesiology
Nephrology	Emergency medicine
Neurology	Nuclear medicine
Pulmonary disease	Pathology
Rheumatology	Physical medicine and rehabilitation
Geriatric medicine	Preventive medicine
Pediatrics	Radiology
Psychiatry	

tasks for physicians, including patient interviews and examinations, treatment of minor illness, and patient education and counseling; some states allow nurses to prescribe medications. Nurses may have Associate Degrees in Nursing (ADNs) obtained from 2-year junior or community colleges, diplomas from 2- to 3-year nursing programs offered by some hospitals and private schools, or Bachelor of Science in Nursing (BSN) degrees from 4-year colleges and universities. Graduates from all three programs are eligible for licensure as registered nurses (RNs); continuing licensure is often contingent on completion of continuing nursing education requirements. Nurse administrations, educators, researchers, clinical specialists, and practitioners usually have master's or doctoral degrees. Nurses may specialize in more than 38 categories based on disease states, patient age, and acuity of illness. Certification is available for some of these specialties. For example, nurses can be certified in critical care and are then entitled to use the designation *Certified Critical Care Registered Nurse* (CCRN) in their titles.

Physician Assistants. Physician assistants (PAs) perform many routine tasks for physicians, such as patient interviews and examinations, treatment of minor illness, and patient education and counseling; PAs can prescribe medications in many states. PAs may have certificates, associate degrees, or master's degrees. Most states require graduates of accredited programs to pass certifying examinations. Those who pass the examination may use the designation *Physician Assistant-Certified* (PA-C). Continuing licensure is contingent on completion of continuing education requirements; recertification examinations must be passed periodically.

THE HEALTH CARE TEAM

The health care team consists of all health care professionals who have responsibility for patient care plus the patient. Although all members of the health care team interact directly with the patient, they rarely meet as a group; instead, information and recommendations are exchanged through written documentation. Verbal information exchange and recommendations occur on a less formal basis.

All members of the health care team contribute their profession's unique knowledge and skills. Pharmacists, the "drug expert" on the team, help teams develop, implement, and monitor the therapeutic regimen and provide drug information and educational services for the patient and team.

Students have a unique role on the health care team. Students represent their profession and are expected to carry out their professional responsibilities under the direct supervision of licensed professionals. For example, pharmacy students are expected to provide patient-focused care under the direct supervision of a licensed pharmacy preceptor. The degree of autonomy and ability to prospectively influence the health care team gradually develop with experience. Although the types of experiences students have vary with the patient care environment, the professional responsibilities remain the same.

THE MEDICAL TEAM

Teaching hospitals are the primary training sites for most health care professionals. Heath care services in teaching hospitals are structured around medical teaching teams composed of physicians, medical students, and depending on the hospital, other health care professionals (Box 1-7). Medical teams, organized to provide a structured training environment for physicians, are responsible for the care of patients located in distinct areas of the hospital (e.g., the cardiology unit) or for patients who are not necessarily located in a geographically distinct area (e.g., infectious disease). The team may provide consultative services in a medical subspecialty (e.g., dermatology) or be identified with a specific physician group practice. The medical team functions as a unit, with the division of labor and the responsibility of each member delegated according to the status of each individual. The team is structured so that each team member receives guidance from a more experienced physician. The team is the focus for group teaching and decision-making discussions. Most trainees spend about 4 weeks with any specific team. Physician team members

---

BOX 1-7

Medical Team Composition in Teaching Hospitals

TYPICAL TEAM MEMBERS	OTHER TEAM MEMBERS
Attending physician	Medical ethicist
Senior or junior medical resident	Nurse
Intern	Occupational therapist
Senior medical student	Pharmacist
Junior medical student	Respiratory therapist
	Social worker
	Students (dental, nursing, pharmacy)

include, in order of seniority, the attending physician, fellows, residents, and medical students.

Attending Physician.   The attending physician is the senior physician on the medical team. The attending physician assumes responsibility for all patients assigned to the team and provides guidance and direction to team members. During team rounds, the attending physician leads the team through the decision-making process, helps the team make decisions regarding patient care, and evaluates the performance of individual team members. Patient presentations may take place in a conference room, in the hallway outside of the patent's room, or in the patients' room. The attending physician spends a short portion of the day with the team and is available for consultation (usually by telephone) throughout the rest of the day, 24-hours a day, 7 days a week.

Fellows.   Medical fellows are physicians who have completed residency training and have elected to continue their training in a research-oriented fellowship program. Fellows work closely with the attending physician and have fewer direct patient care responsibilities than residents. Fellows teach the more junior members of the team. In some fellowship programs, fellows are responsible for performing specific invasive procedures such as arterial line placement, bronchoscopy, and endoscopy. Research-intensive, multiyear fellowship programs in medical subspecialty areas such as gastroenterology, cardiology, neurology, and pulmonary medicine are available at many major teaching hospitals.

Residents.   Medical residents are physicians who have graduated from medical schools and are in structured and supervised residency training programs.

First-year residents (sometimes designated as *postgraduate year 1, PGY1,* or *PG1*) are known as *interns.* Internal medicine internships of at least 1 year often are required before the resident moves on to more specialized training in areas such as surgery and psychiatry. The intern year also is the first of several years of training for physicians interested in practicing internal medicine. Interns, who are licensed physicians, have an intensive year of training, with frequent night call and direct responsibility for the care of a variety of inpatients and outpatients. Interns typically spend 1-month periods gaining experience in a variety of internal medical services such as general medicine, emergency room services, and intensive care services. In addition, interns usually have set clinic hours and see a variety of outpatients over the course of the year.

Second-year internal medical residents (sometimes designated as *postgraduate year 2, PGY2,* or *PG2*) also are known as *junior admitting residents* (JARs). *Third-year* medical residents (*postgraduate year 3, PGY3,* or *PG3*), also known as *senior admitting residents* (SARs), are in the final year of 3-year internal medicine residency programs. The senior medical resident sets the daily team rounding schedule, prioritizes the work schedule, coordinates the team work, supervises the interns, supervises and works closely with the medical students on the team, and consults with the attending physician. Residents have frequent night call and direct responsibility for a variety of inpatients and outpatients.

The *chief medical resident* is a senior medical resident who, in addition to the usual resident responsibilities, has administrative responsibility for various aspects of the residency program, such as scheduling rotations and vacations and organizing and overseeing seminars and other education programs. The chief medical resident position is competitive; typically one or two residents per year are selected for this position.

Medical Students.   Although medical students get some experience examining and interviewing patients in the first or second year of medical school, clinical clerkships usually start in the third year of medical school. Third-year medical students, known as *junior medical students*, spend part of the year in the patient care environment in month-long rotations such as internal medicine, surgery, obstetrics and gynecology, and pediatric services. Their patient workloads are limited to a small number of patients, and medical school faculty and more experienced team members closely supervise them. Senior medical students, also known as *externs*, are in the last year of medical school. Depending on the medical school curriculum, senior medical students may spend all or part of the last year of medical school in a variety of selective or elective rotations. Externs have more patient care responsibilities than do junior medical students but less than interns or other residents.

The medical team, depending on institution-specific policies, may include a variety of other health care professionals. Some pharmacists provide patient care services to specified patient population (e.g., oncology, critical care, nutrition, transplant, nephrology) and are considered integral members of the medical team. Pharmacy residents, fellows, and students often are assigned to specific internal medicine teams for part of their experiential training. Nurse practitioners may provide patient care services to specific patient populations and attend rounds with the medical team. More commonly, nurse specialists join the medical team as the team discusses specific patients and patient-specific issues. Nursing students may be assigned to medical teams as part of their experiential training. Other health care professionals who may be part of the team or join the medical team on rounds on specific patients include social workers, dietitians, medical ethicists, occupational therapists, physical therapists, and respiratory therapists.

THE INPATIENT ENVIRONMENT

Patients admitted to the hospital are assigned beds on specific floors, wards, or wings according to the specific medical problem (e.g., obstetrics, general medicine, cardiology, orthopedics). The admitting physician evaluates the patient and orders laboratory tests, procedures, diets, and medications. The admitting physician may consult with specialty physicians and other health care professionals, including pharmacists. In a teaching hospital, medical residents, interns, and medical students also evaluate the patient; the physician of record (the resident or intern) generates patient orders and consults with a variety of physicians and other health care professionals regarding patient care.

Nursing services are organized to provide 24-hour nursing coverage for all patients. The number of patients assigned to each nurse depends on the severity of illness or disability and ranges from 1 or more nurses per critically ill patient to 10 or more patients per nurse on other units. Each floor, unit, or ward has a head nurse with administrative responsibility for nursing services. Some hospitals assign each patient to a primary nurse practitioner who determines the nursing care plan for the patient and coordinates patient care.

Medical team rounds usually occur in the morning. Work rounds, led by the medical resident, usually occur early in the morning. During work rounds the patient's progress is briefly reviewed by the resident, intern, or medical student responsible for the patient; the medical team visits each patient. Work rounds allow all members of the team to catch up on the status of each patient and plan for the day's tests, consultations, and other patient care activities.

Attending rounds, led by the attending physician, generally occur after work rounds and are held in conference rooms rather than at the patient's bedside. Newly admitted patients are presented to the attending physician, who leads the discussion of the differential diagnosis and decision-making processes. Other patients may be discussed in detail. Although some teaching takes place during work rounds, most in-depth teaching discussions take place during attending rounds.

Team members spend the rest of the day independently evaluating patients, assessing laboratory and diagnostic test results, documenting patient findings, consulting with other health care providers, and planning for the care of their patients. The team may gather for radiology rounds, during which recent patient radiographs (e.g., chest films, computed tomography scans) are reviewed. At the end of the day the team gathers for sign-out rounds, during which the physician responsible for providing medical coverage in the evening and overnight is briefed about each patient on the service.

THE OUTPATIENT ENVIRONMENT

Physicians and other primary care providers (e.g., physician assistants, nurse practitioners, pharmacists) evaluate outpatients in private offices and clinics. Some clinics provide "first come, first served" walk-in services; most require appointments. The health care professional-patient interaction generally is short (10 to 12 minutes) except for initial patient evaluations, more complex patients, and procedures. Patients are referred to affiliated or freestanding facilities for laboratory and diagnostic procedures such as blood work, radiographs, and scans; the results are sent to the referring health care provider.

THE MEDICAL RECORD

The inpatient medical record, also known as the *chart,* is a legal document that includes sections for hospital-specific admission and insurance information, initial history and physical examination, daily progress notes written by every health care professional who interacts with the patient, consultations, nursing notes, laboratory results, and radiology and surgery reports (Figure 1-2). Most charts include sections for medication orders and other types of orders (e.g., laboratory, dietary, diagnostic procedures) (Table 1-1); some hospitals maintain a separate ordering system. Upon discharge, the medical record is stored in the medical records department and is retrievable by referencing the patent's hospital admission number. Sophisticated computer systems enable all or part of the medical record to be accessed electronically. Access to electronic charts is restricted to authorized health care professionals. Electronic charts contain the same sections and are structured the same as traditional written charts. Access to the chart generally is limited to specific individual or group practice health care professionals.

Many institutions and practices chart in a specified format known as a *problem-oriented medical record,* or *POMR.* The POMR is structured around a prioritized patient problem list. Progress notes and discharge summaries address each patient problem as listed on the patient problem list.

Every page of the medical record, all patient-specific orders, and every page printed from the computerized chart are stamped or printed with a patient identification number. In most hospitals a plastic card that includes the patient's name, race, address, physician, birth date, date of admission, and hospital admission num-

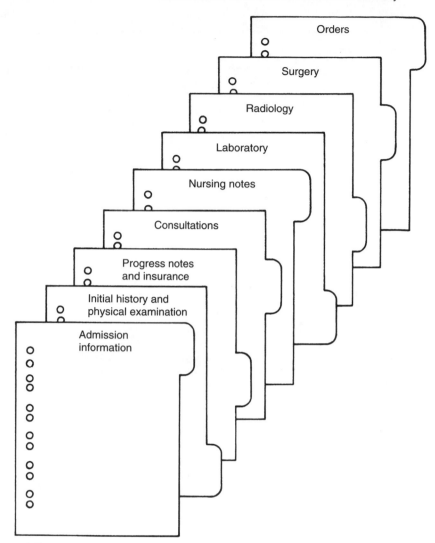

Figure 1-2
Components of the Medical Record.
The medical record contains sections for many types of patient-specific information.

ber is created upon admission. A ward secretary (also known as a *ward clerk*) coordinates the processing of paperwork on a hospital unit or part of a hospital unit. Some large units have two or more ward secretaries.

The outpatient medical record or chart contains the same type of information as the inpatient chart with the exception of the admitting data, physician orders, admission history and physical examination, and medication administration sections. Outpatient charts are used more to document patient-specific encounters and data than to communicate with other health care professionals. Therefore outpatient chart documentation is limited compared with inpatient charts.

TABLE 1-1

Medical Record Content

Section	Type of Information
Admitting data	Name, address, date of birth, insurance, next of kin
Consent forms	Consent for surgery, procedures, research studies
Physician orders	Medication, dietary, and laboratory orders
Flow sheets and graphic charts	24-hour charts of blood pressure, heart rate, respiratory rate, temperature, and fluid intake and output
Progress notes	Daily physician notes, nursing shift notes, consultant notes
Laboratory data	Blood chemistries, arterial blood gases, cultures and sensitivities, histopathology reports
Diagnostic procedures	Radiology and other diagnostic procedures reports
Consults	Consultant assessments and recommendations
Operating room reports	Preoperative checklist, anesthesia record, graphic records of vital signs, description of events during surgery
Admission history and physical examination	Initial history and physical examination
Medication administration record	Date, time, dose of medications administered; names and initial of nurses who administered medications; lists of all ordered medications
Miscellaneous	Emergency room record

THE HEALTH CARE DELIVERY SYSTEM

The health care delivery system in the United States has evolved over the past several decades from a system that held individuals financially responsible for all aspects of their health care to the current system, which advocates equal access and financial support for all components of health care, including sophisticated and technologically advanced health care, for all individuals. Many Americans believe that access to medical care is a national right. However, the financial burden of this philosophy has stimulated considerable debate regarding the best way to use limited societal health care resources.

The health care system is a complex system influenced and controlled by a variety of private and federal factors. Some early attempts at public support of needy individuals date back to the early 1700s in colonial America; however, the prevailing attitude of the time was that individuals, not society, pay for health care. Health care professionals and institutions were free to charge "customary, prevailing, and reasonable" fees for services; patients paid for private insurance or whatever they could afford to purchase if not covered by insurance. The health care system thus evolved to meet the needs of those who could afford to purchase expensive and inclusive service. Unfortunately, this type of health care system excluded portions of society. The federal government has had to gradually assume financial and regulatory con-

TABLE 1-2	

Public Health Policy Development

Date	Issue
1930s-1940s	Limited support for special patient populations
1940s-1950s	Support for research, facilities, and training
1960s	Broadened health care coverage
1970s	Infrastructure support
1980s-1990s	Cost, quality, and outcomes

From Kissick WL: *Trans Stud Coll Phys Phila* 11:187-200, 1989.

trol of larger portions of the system.[3] Public health policy evolved from a focus on limited support for special patient populations in the 1930s and 1940s to interest in cost, quality, and outcomes in the 1990s (Table 1-2).

Many health care issues remain unresolved. The most pressing of these is how to decrease costs while maintaining high-quality health care. Inequities in the health care system are significant; more than one fourth of the population is inadequately insured or completely without health insurance.[4,5] The number of unoccupied hospital beds is large, increasing the competition for traditional and new hospital services (e.g., wellness clinics, fitness centers). Regional oversupply and undersupply of physicians and other health care professionals exists. The cost of medical malpractice to both the physician and the health care system is high. Defensive medicine accounts for an estimated 15% of the total U.S. expenditures for physician services.[6] Finally, the roles of pharmacists, nurses, and physician assistants are still evolving, and many questions regarding authority and responsibility for patient care remain unanswered.

SELF-ASSESSMENT QUESTIONS

1. Which of the following is *not* an outcome included in the definition of pharmaceutical care?
   a. Cure of disease
   b. Elimination or reduction of symptoms
   c. Arresting or slowing of disease processes
   d. Prevention of disease or symptoms
   e. Reduction of health care costs

2. Skills required for patient-centered pharmacy practice include which of the following?
   a. Therapeutic planning and monitoring skills
   b. Physical assessment skills
   c. Communication skills
   d. All of the above
   e. None of the above

3. To be eligible for board certification, pharmacists need which of the following?
   a. A Doctor of Pharmacy degree
   b. Advanced education and training or equivalent experience
   c. A postgraduate residency
   d. At least 5 years of work experience
   e. Three letters of recommendation

4. Board certification for pharmacists is *not* available in which one of the following areas?
   a. Pharmacokinetics
   b. Pharmacotherapy
   c. Nutrition
   d. Nuclear pharmacy
   e. Psychiatric pharmacy practice

5. Pharmacy fellowship programs prepare pharmacists to become which of the following?
   a. Educators
   b. Practitioners
   c. Business leaders
   d. Researchers
   e. Administrators

6. Outpatient health care settings include all of the following *except*:
   a. Clinics
   b. Day surgery units
   c. Rehabilitation centers
   d. Emergency rooms
   e. Private offices

7. Veterans Administration hospitals are which of the following?
   a. Public hospitals
   b. Private hospitals
   c. Federal hospitals
   d. City hospitals
   e. State hospitals

8. Which of the following team members prioritizes and coordinates the work of the medical team?
   a. Attending physician
   b. Second- or third-year resident
   c. Fellow
   d. Senior medical student
   e. Junior medical student

9. In teaching hospitals, most in-depth teaching discussions take place during which of the following activities?
   a. Sign-out rounds
   b. Work rounds
   c. Radiology rounds
   d. Attending rounds
   e. Shift change

10. Unresolved health care issues include which of the following?
    a. How to decrease the cost of quality health care
    b. The imbalance between supply and distribution of physician services
    c. The role of clinical pharmacists, nurse practitioners, and PAs
    d. All of the above
    e. None of the above

References

1. Hepler CD, Strand LM: Opportunities and responsibilities in pharmaceutical care, *Am J Hosp Pharm* 47:533-543, 1990.
2. Definitions of pharmacy residencies and fellowships, *Am J Hosp Pharm* 44:1142-1144, 1987.
3. Kissick WL: The evolution of American health policy, *Trans Stud Coll Phys Phila* 11:187-200, 1989.
4. Orford RR: Reflections on the Canadian and American health-care systems, *Mayo Clin Proc* 66:203-206, 1991.
5. Davies NE, Felder LH: Applying brakes to the runaway American health care system, JAMA 263:73-76, 1990.
6. Reynolds RA, Rizzo JA, Gonzalez ML: The cost of medical professional liability, JAMA 257:2776-2781, 1987.

Communication Skills for the Pharmacist

CHAPTER 2

Learning Objectives

- Describe how to promote two-way communication with patients and health care professionals.
- Identify common barriers to verbal communication and describe ways to overcome each barrier.
- List at least six guidelines for documenting patient information in the medical record.
- State how to convey respect for patients.
- Identify patient situations that affect patient-pharmacist communication and suggest ways to deal with each situation.
- State how to communicate effectively with physicians, nurses, and other pharmacists.
- Identify skills for effective teaching, platform and poster presentations, and media interviews.

The ability to communicate clearly and effectively with patients, family members, physicians, nurses, pharmacists, and other health care professionals is an important skill. Some pharmacists are skilled communicators, comfortable with all types of people; other pharmacists find it difficult to communicate with health care providers in perceived or actual positions of authority or with patients from different socioeconomic or ethnic backgrounds. Fortunately, communication skills can be learned. One incentive for improving communication skills is that pharmacists with excellent communication skills and average pharmacy databases are more likely to be successful than pharmacists with poor communication skills and excellent pharmacy databases. Another incentive is that the inability to communicate effectively may harm patients. Poor communication between a pharmacist and a patient may result in an inaccurate patient medication history and inappropriate therapeutic decisions; may contribute to patient confusion, disinterest, and noncompliance; and may add to a patient's frustration with the health care system. Poor communication between pharmacists and physicians, pharmacists and nurses, and pharmacists and pharmacists may harm patients if important information is not exchanged in an appropriate and timely manner.

VERBAL COMMUNICATION SKILLS

Essential verbal communication skills include the ability to listen, understand, and respond to what people say (active listening) and the ability to interpret nonverbal communication and respond in a way that encourages continued interaction (evaluation).

ACTIVE LISTENING

Focus on the patient, family member, or health care professional. Make that person feel like the center of attention. Convey an open, relaxed, and unhurried attitude. Set aside all professional and personal distractions and really focus on the person. Prevent or minimize interruptions (e.g., beepers, telephone calls, consultations).

Focus on the person and how he or she communicates (Figure 2-1). The tone and modulation of voice and number and placement of pauses may disclose how the person feels and may provide clues regarding the reliability of the patient-provided information. People who respond with a low level of energy, flat affect, and monotone voice may be depressed. People who respond to questions tentatively and hesitantly may be unreliable. Pauses may indicate that the person needs time to recall the information or find the right words or that the person is censoring the response or preparing to lie.

OBSERVATION AND ASSESSMENT

Effective two-way communication requires continual observation and assessment of how the other person is communicating. Body language and gestures provide important clues for the pharmacist, as well as the patient and health care provider.

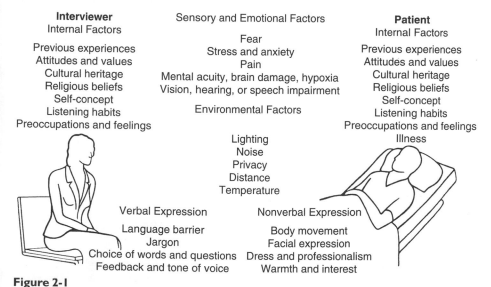

Figure 2-1

Factors Influencing Communication.

Communication is affected by the integration of patient and pharmacist internal factors; sensory, emotional, and environmental factors; and verbal and nonverbal expression. (From Wilkins RL, Sheldon RL, Krider SJ: *Clinical assessment in respiratory care*, ed 2, St Louis, 1990, Mosby.)

Sit or stand at eye level, maintain eye contact, and use a focused body posture to convey interest and attentiveness. Sitting or standing at eye level or lower projects a nonthreatening, equalizing body position that facilitates open communication. Be physically close enough to the patient, family member, or health care professional for clear and comprehensible communication but do not intrude on the other person's personal space. Invasion of personal space induces discomfort and may be perceived as physically threatening; in either case, communication is compromised.

Be aware of nonverbal messages. Certain gestures and postures provide clues regarding the other persons' feelings (Table 2-1), although the clues are not always reliable. Change tactics to reengage the person if their body language indicates closure to communication.

BARRIERS TO VERBAL COMMUNICATION

Physical Barriers.   Communication across or through physical barriers is extremely difficult. Physical barriers commonly encountered in community pharmacies include the large countertops and display areas behind which many pharmacists work, windows with security bars and protective glass, drive-through windows that isolate the pharmacist from the patient, and the elevated pharmacy work area that accentuates the pharmacist's position of authority and places the patient in an inferior position.

Hospital and other institutional pharmacists have fewer physical barriers to contend with but have the additional problem of communicating with patients who are in bed. Patients in bed are easily intimidated by people standing over them. Interviews may be strained or limited depending on the patient's level of discomfort. Make sure all conversations take place face to face at or below the patient's eye level.

Lack of Privacy.   Lack of privacy is a common communication barrier. Although lack of privacy often is identified as a barrier to effective communication with patients, it also is an important barrier when communicating with other health care professionals. Breach of privacy is possible whenever patient information is discussed. Do not discuss or debate nonspecific or specific patient data or health care issues in public areas such as hallways, walkways, elevators, cafeterias, libraries, and parking lots. Do not discuss patient-specific information with family or friends.

TABLE 2-1

Body Language

Gesture or Posture	Implication
Steepling of the hands	Confidence
Raising the hand	Desire to interrupt
Shifting body position	Desire to interrupt
Crossed arms	Shutting out the other person
Leaning toward the speaker	Receptiveness
Raising the hands and then letting them fall limply	Hopelessness
Frequent throat clearing	Disagreement

Lack of privacy is a common problem in most health care settings. Few community pharmacies have private counseling areas. Most hospitalized patients have at least one roommate; three or more patients may share some hospital wards. The lack of privacy makes the voicing of personal concerns and the exchange of accurate and complete information difficult for many patients. Given a choice, patients may withhold potentially embarrassing personal information or avoid asking potentially embarrassing or "stupid" questions if they think the conversation may be overheard.

Provide as much privacy as possible. Ideally, converse with patients and discuss patient-specific information with other health care professionals in private counseling or consultation rooms. If physically separate space is not available, converse in a space that is as private as possible. In community pharmacies, converse with patients in a corner of the pharmacy away from the cash register, drop off windows, and pick up windows. In hospitals and other institutions, create a sense of privacy by closing the door to the room and pulling the curtain around the bed. Ambulatory institutionalized patients may be able to walk to nearby conference rooms, private consultation rooms, or vacant waiting rooms.

The Telephone.   The telephone is an important communication tool used to communicate with patients, patient family members, physicians, nurses, other pharmacists, and other health care professionals. Speak clearly, listen carefully, be organized, and state facts clearly and calmly.

Those initiating the telephone conversation should identify themselves by name and state the purpose of the call. For example, when calling a physician office, say "Hello. This is Joan Arnold. I'm the pharmacist working with Mrs. Johnson. I have a question about Mrs. Johnson's diabetic drug regimen. May I please speak with Dr. Rivers?" Be prepared to repeat the request several times before being connected to the right person. Stay patient and tolerate and expect to spend some time waiting on hold.

When answering telephone calls, identify yourself and ask for the caller's identity. Make every effort to deal with the call immediately; avoid putting the other person on hold. If too busy to speak with the caller at that moment, explain the situation to the caller immediately and arrange to call back at a mutually convenient time rather than placing the person on hold. Most telephone calls are directly related to patient care and need to be dealt with as soon as possible. Interruptive telephone calls should be dealt with as unhurriedly and professionally as possible.

Pharmacists sometimes receive telephone calls from angry and upset patients, patient family members, nurses, physicians, and other health care professionals. The best way to deal with these types of calls is to stay calm, listen to what the person has to say, clarify the issue, and then handle the problem as calmly and coolly as possible. Nothing is accomplished if both parties let their emotions rule the interactions.

WRITTEN COMMUNICATION SKILLS

Pharmacists must be able to accurately and effectively document patient information in the patient medical record, document patient information in pharmacy medication profiles and other pharmacy records, and correspond with patients and other health care professionals. Many pharmacists routinely document written drug information responses; this skill is discussed in Chapter 9.

The patient medical record is the primary written communication tool for all health care professionals. Health care professionals who care for patients in the inpatient setting write daily progress notes in patient charts. Professionals in the outpatient setting write progress notes after each patient visit. Writing in a patient medical record (charting) is a privilege granted by each institution or organization to individual health care professionals. Many institutions and organizations grant pharmacists charting privileges, although this practice is far from universal.

The medical record ordinarily is used to document and communicate information about the patient's progress; to assess, usually retrospectively, the quality and appropriateness of patient care; and to document patient care activities and services for remuneration. Health care professionals must adhere to legal, ethical, and professional standards when documenting patient information (Box 2-1). Black ink is photocopied more clearly than other colors and is recommended just in case the patient record has to be photocopied (e.g., subpoenaed for a legal hearing or forwarded to health care professionals outside the institution or practice). Clear photocopies reduce the risk of misreading or misinterpreting the documented information. Clear and legible handwriting is important. Errors are dealt with by crossing out the error with one line and initialing the error (e.g., ~~misteak~~[RS] mistake). This format clearly documents the error and identifies the individual who changed the record. Products that paint over typewritten or handwritten information are not used on legal documents because they hide the error and could be used by anyone at anytime to change the record.

Document factual information and restrict assessments and judgments to those appropriate for pharmacists. For example, a pharmacist may learn during a patient medication history interview that the patient drinks a fifth of whiskey and a six-pack of beer daily. It is appropriate to document the facts but inappropriate to label the patient an alcoholic.

Every note in the patient medical record contains a descriptive heading (e.g., clinical pharmacy, pharmacokinetics, nutrition support, attending, cardiology consult), the date and time the note was written, patient-specific data and other information, and the signature and title of the health care professional. The heading identifies the type of information found in the note and enables individuals using the chart to scan the pages quickly when searching for specific information. The date and time are important details that put the information in context with other patient-related data and information. For example, a pharmacist may assess a patient and make drug and dosing recommendations before that day's laboratory results are available. Knowing the time of the recommendation allows the other members of the health care team to accept or reject the recommendation in context of the most up-to-date patient data. The content of the note is organized using a SOAP format (Subjective,

---

BOX 2-1

Guidelines for Writing Medical Record Notes

1. Use black ink.
2. Write clearly and legibly.
3. Label notes with specific descriptive headings.
4. Provide the date and time on the notes.
5. Document the facts and avoid making unsubstantiated judgments.
6. Organize the information using the SOAP or freestyle format.
7. Sign the note with name and title.

*O*bjective, *A*ssessment, *P*lan) or a freestyle format. The SOAP format is a universally recognized structured format (see Chapter 7), whereas a freestyle format has no accepted organizational structure. The health care professional writing the note signs the note. Documents or notes written by students and other nonlicensed trainees are cosigned by the licensed professional who is supervising the nonlicensed individual.

Most institutions, outpatient clinics, and individual practices are transitioning from handwritten charts to electronic charts. Data are entered using bedside computer terminals or any computer in the system, eliminating "competition" for the written chart. Electronic charts limit access to confidential patient information to individuals with approved passwords but expand access to the charted information by allowing entry from any computer within the system. The computer automatically labels the data with the date and time and the name of the person linked to the password.

INTEGRATION

COMMUNICATING WITH PATIENTS

Effective communication between pharmacists and patients or family members is extremely important to pharmaceutical care. Ineffective communication leads to confusion and misunderstanding and may contribute to inappropriate decisions regarding drug therapy.

Patient Titles.   Unfortunately, most health care professionals automatically address patients by their first names, even when meeting patients for the first time.[1] Some patients take offense at being addressed by their first names, especially if they are much older than the health care professional. Health care professionals who automatically expect patients to address them by title compound the offense. This expectation puts the patient in an unequal and inferior position and is a throwback to the days of paternalistic health care attitudes. Some patients offended by being addressed by their first names may openly express their displeasure. Other patients may be so put off by this behavior that they are unwilling to engage in productive conversation.

Common courtesy dictates that patients be addressed by appropriate title (e.g., Mr., Mrs., Ms., Rev., Dr.). However, use the correct title. Do not assume that all adult women are married or, if married, wish to be addressed as "Mrs." Conversely, do not assume that all adult women, married or single, want to be addressed as "Ms." The best way to avoid confusion is to ask each patient how he or she wants to be addressed. Saying "Hello. My name is Dr. Smith. Do you wish to be called Ms. or Mrs. Sandborne or would you prefer to be called Elizabeth?" requires very little time or effort. This approach conveys a sense of respect for the patient, allows the patient to express their preference, and indicates to the patient how to address the health care professional. The one exception to this approach is in addressing disoriented, confused, or sedated patients; these patients usually respond better to their first names than to their titles.

Respect for the Patient.   Display a genuine respect for the patient. Respond to the patient as a person, not a prescription or case (e.g., "The asthma patient in room 1012"). Maintain a professional relationship and avoid exchanging personal information and confidences with the patient, remembering, "An interview is a conversation with a purpose rather than a conversation with a potential friend."[2]

Respect for the patient is conveyed by acknowledging, without judgment, patient-specific attributes that may be different from the pharmacist's value system or even offensive to the pharmacist. Attributes such as smoking, excessive drinking, use of illicit drugs, self-destructive behaviors, nonadherence to prescribed regimens, deficient hygiene, and gross obesity may be offensive but must be dealt with nonjudgmentally. Other patient-specific traits such as beliefs in folk physiology or use of alternative remedies or unorthodox medical treatments also must be acknowledged without judgment. Pharmacists also must be able to acknowledge differences in socioeconomic backgrounds and ethnic origins without passing judgment.

Respect for the patient is conveyed by pharmacist's attitude (Box 2-2). Arrange adequate time for patient interaction and minimize interruptions from phone calls, beepers, and other patients or health care professionals. Introduce yourself, obtain permission to interact with the patient, and explain the purpose of the interaction. Explain who will see the information obtained by the pharmacist and how the information will be used. Pharmacy students need to clearly identify themselves as students and explain who will see information obtained during the student-patient interaction and the way in which the information will be used (e.g., for teaching purposes, for patient care, for research).

The environment established by the pharmacist conveys respect for the patient. The physical environment should be clean, neat, and well organized. Make sure the patient is as comfortable as possible and provide as much privacy as possible (refer to the Barriers to Communication section later in this chapter). Remove as many barriers to communication as possible (refer to the Barriers to Communication section later in this chapter). Note taking during the patient interaction is acceptable but should not control the interaction.

Questioning Techniques. The pharmacist, not the patient, controls the patient-pharmacist interaction. The pharmacist controls the interaction by controlling the types of questions asked and the time allowed for patient response. Controlling the interaction does not mean, however, that the pharmacist should fire off a rapid sequence of yes/no questions or abruptly cut off patient response. Questioning skills improve as the pharmacist gains experience interacting with a variety of patients, including pleasant and not so pleasant, cooperative and uncooperative, verbose and recalcitrant, and interested and disinterested patients.

BOX 2-2

Behavioral Checklist

Be relaxed, confident, and comfortable.
Show interest in the patient.
Maintain objectivity.
Be nonjudgmental.
Be sincere and honest.
Maintain control of the interview.

From Zakus GE et al: J Med Ed 51:323-331, 1976.

Early in the interview, ask open-ended questions that allow patients to talk freely about their medications and concerns. This technique clues the patient that the pharmacist is interested in what he or she has to say and gives the pharmacist feedback regarding the patient's level of knowledge and ability to communicate this information. A good initial question for both acute care and chronic care patients is, "What medications are you currently taking?" Use minimal facilitators such as "yes," "uh huh," and "what else?" and provide nonverbal encouragement by smiling and nodding when appropriate. Give the patient time to answer. Some patients can provide well-organized and detailed information without much additional direction; however, other patients ramble and shift to nonrelated topics. Some patients cannot provide any information without specific targeted questions. Some patients have told their story so many times that they automatically recite their story or what they think the pharmacist wants to hear without focusing on the pharmacist's questions.

Ask directed and structured questions after the patient has presented his or her story or has begun to stray from the initial question. Narrow the focus of the question as appropriate. Discuss one topic at a time and avoid asking leading questions, multiple questions, and yes/no questions. Simple yes/no questions are useful screening questions but inhibit the patient's flow of information when used excessively.

Take time during the patient interaction to summarize the information provided by the patient. This lets the patient know what the pharmacist has learned, gives the pharmacist a chance to verify the information, and ensures that the patient and pharmacist are in agreement. Frequent summaries also let the pharmacist identify and correct any discrepancies in the patient's story.

Close the patient-pharmacist interaction by providing a final summary of the information obtained from the patient. Let the patient make any final clarifications or add additional information. End the interaction by thanking the patient pleasantly and say "good-bye."

Patient Instruction.   Pharmacists tend to consider the prescription label the primary communication tool between the pharmacist and the patient. However, optimal patient interaction requires more than this one-way communication tool. Several communication objectives for patient instruction have been identified,[4] including identification of the patient's needs, control of the timing and amount of information provided during each interaction, determination of patient-specific objectives, and assessment of patient learning. For example, the pharmacist cannot assume that asthmatic patients use metered-dose inhalers correctly or know how to monitor their lung function with a peak flow meter. Question such patients to determine their depth of knowledge and degree of understanding; then develop a plan for patient education. Plan to convey drug-specific information over several sessions and provide such patients with written information to reinforce the verbal information.

Assess patient needs in the context of the patient's emotional status, educational background, and intellectual ability. Some patients want to know everything about their medication. Other patients do not want to know anything. Balance the patient's desire for information with the need for information. At the end of the interaction determine the depth of the patient's learning and retention in a non-threatening manner. Ask the patient to summarize or repeat the information discussed. Over time and through repeated interaction, the pharmacist can convey a large amount of drug-specific information and help the patient successfully manage the medication regimen.

TABLE 2-2

Commonly Misunderstood Terms

Term	Meaning
Allergic	A response stimulated by an allergen
Antibiotic	A drug that inhibits the growth of microorganisms
Antihistamine	A medication that blocks the action of histamine
Controlled substance	A medication with addictive potential
Cough suppressant	A medication that reduces cough
Decongestant	A medication that reduces congestion
Diuretic	A medication that increases the amount of urine
Generic	The nonproprietary name for a medication
Hypertension	High arterial blood pressure
Inflammation	A complex pathologic process that affects blood vessels and tissues
Oral	Relating to the mouth
Over-the-counter (OTC) drugs	Nonprescription medications
Third-party payers	Organizations that pay health care bills

From Shaughnessy AF: Am Pharm NS28:38-42, 1988.

Medical Jargon.   Avoid medical jargon when communicating with patients. This can be challenging, but pharmacists must be able to translate commonly used pharmacy and medical terms into lay terminology. Results from a study evaluating patient understanding of commonly used pharmacy terms (Table 2-2) indicated that many patients did not understand these terms; in fact, many patients interpreted these terms quite differently than they were intended.[5] For example, some patients thought the term *diuretic* meant a medication for diarrhea or concerned the diet or diabetes; some patients thought the term *generic* meant synthetic or not as good or thought the term concerned the elderly.

Patients misinterpret even commonly used medical terms. For example, the term *hypertension* has multiple meanings to patients. Some patients think it means hyperactive or nervous. Some cultures use the term *high blood* to indicate hypertension and *low blood* to indicate anemia. Other terms, such as *angina, divided dose, anticoagulant, sublingual, subcutaneous, intravenous,* and *dyspnea,* may have no meaning whatsoever for the typical patient.

The best way to avoid miscommunication and confusion is to speak in plain English and use concrete and specific references. Provide many opportunities for patients to ask questions. Be especially sensitive to the needs of nonnative English speakers who may be confused by American slang or cultural references. Use translators for patients who do not speak or understand English. Be aware that some patients, especially those with chronic disease, frequent contacts with the health care system, or a health care background, may have sophisticated pharmacy and medical vocabularies and may be offended by the use of simplified lay terminology.

Special Situations.   Pharmacists must be able to communicate with patients who are unable or unwilling to communicate along generally accepted societal norms. The patient's situation or attitude may compromise communication. Some patients are so stressed by acute or chronic illnesses that they do not adhere to common rules of courtesy. Communication with such patients may be extremely difficult. Differences in ethnic, social, and educational backgrounds may make communication between the patient and pharmacist difficult. The pharmacist, not the patient, is responsible for recognizing the special situation and having the skills and flexibility necessary to ensure appropriate and effective communication.

Embarrassing Situations. Most patients find discussions related to sex, intimate body parts, and bodily functions embarrassing (Box 2-3).[6] Many female community pharmacists have had the experience of watching men loiter in the pharmacy until they can ask a male clerk about condoms. Asking male pharmacists about the application of vaginal creams or suppositories embarrasses many female patients. Some patients are so embarrassed by such situations that they deliberately avoid asking for help, choosing to remain uninformed rather than risk the embarrassment (Figure 2-2).

To deal with these situations, be aware of what may be potentially embarrassing and be ready to bring up the subject if the patient has difficulty doing so. Converse with the patient in as private an environment as possible. Be sensitive to clues that suggest potential embarrassment and communicate with patients in a respectful, professional manner.

Clues to a patent's embarrassment include avoidance of eye contact, blushing, stammering, closed body language, and excessive nervous small talk about unrelated matters (e.g., the weather, sports). Project a professional demeanor and put the patient at ease by discussing the issue in a straightforward, scientifically appropriate manner. Humor, which may temporarily relieve tension, may make the patient more embarrassed and should be avoided. Use anatomically correct terms instead of slang. Give patients many opportunities to express their feelings.

Mute Patients. Muteness from endotracheal intubation, tracheostomy, or damage to the vocal cords or trachea from disease or trauma can be extremely frustrating

---

BOX 2-3

Potentially Embarrassing Situations

Asking about drug-induced sexual dysfunction
Asking for any of the following:
    Hemorrhoid products
    Enema supplies
    Douche supplies
    Ostomy supplies
    Birth control products
Discussing any of the following:
    Drug or substance abuse
    Alcoholism
    Obesity
    Illiteracy
    Constipation
    Incontinence
    Noncompliance

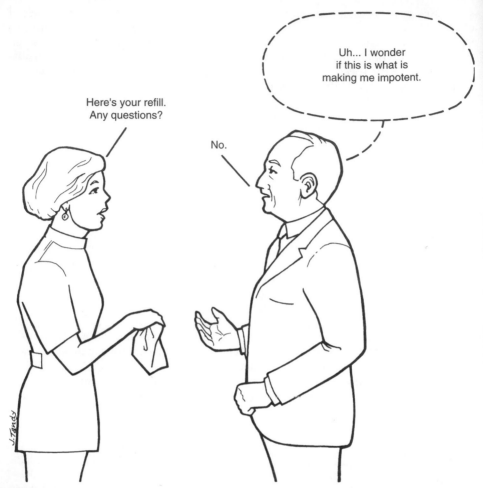

Figure 2-2
Embarrassing Situations.
Some patients are so embarrassed by their situations that they choose silence rather than public disclosure.

for patients. The situation can be equally frustrating for pharmacists, who rely on verbal information from patients when obtaining patient information and monitoring response to therapy. Written communication and point and spell letter boards can be time-consuming but often are the only means for two-way communication. Encourage these techniques and allow sufficient time for adequate communication. In addition, maintain your end of the conversation and do not limit your verbal responses just because the patient is mute.

Elderly Patients.   Elderly patients have special needs.[7,8] Elderly patients may have impaired hearing and vision. The hearing loss associated with aging is characterized by loss of ability to distinguish between high-frequency sounds, making it difficult for patients to distinguish between conversational tones and background noises. Visual changes associated with aging include loss of accommodation, cataracts, reduced peripheral vision, and problems distinguishing some colors. Elderly patients may be sensitive to harsh, glaring lights and highly reflective surfaces. They may not be able to read prescription labels and other printed material or distinguish among similarly shaped dosage formulations.

Take the time to engage elderly patients in unhurried conversation. Speak slowly, distinctly, and avoid youth-oriented vernacular or slang. Treat elderly patients with respect. Do not assume that every elderly person has impaired hearing. Speak directly to the patient and do not assume the patient is incompetent or that the person accompanying the patient is a caregiver or guardian. Use large-print labels and printed materials and reinforce written information with verbal communication. Touching the patient lightly on the arm or shoulder may reassure the patient and reinforce the context of the conversation.

Pediatric Patients. Communicate directly with the pediatric patient as well as with the parent or guardian; do not assume that children have nothing to contribute to their health care. Even young children can understand why they are taking a medication and can begin to develop a professional relationship with the pharmacist. However, information must be age appropriate. For example, communication with young children may be as simple as telling them why they are going to take the medication (e.g., "This medication will help you breathe better"). In-depth information exchange is appropriate for many preteens and teenagers. Direct communication with preteens and teenagers who have chronic disease for which they follow chronic medication regimens is especially important. Preteens and teenagers exert considerable control over their lives and need to understand how to use their medications.

Physically Challenged Patients. Physically challenged patients often have to deal with multiple communication barriers.[9] Pharmacists, like most members of society, often have a hard time focusing on the person in the wheelchair or seeing the patient behind the prosthetic device. Many people falsely assume that physical disabilities are linked with mental disabilities. In addition to these perceptual difficulties, some physical disabilities leave the patient with limited or garbled speech, making it difficult for the patient to express himself or herself. Other disabilities impair a patient's vision or hearing.

Communicating with physically challenged patients is no different than communicating with physically able patients. Engage the patient in unhurried conversation and give the patient ample time to respond. Speak directly to the patient and do not assume that the patient is incompetent. Do not assume that the person accompanying the patient is the patient's caregiver. Do not stare at the patient or avoid eye contact and do not physically assist the patient (e.g., push a wheelchair, guide a blind patient) unless invited to do so by the patient.

Mentally Retarded Patients. Communicate clearly and directly with mentally retarded patients and do not assume that the patients are incapable of participating in their health care. Look beyond the disability and deal directly with the patient. However, communicate clearly and directly with the patient's caregiver. Many degrees of mental retardation are possible; be flexible enough to assess the level to which each patient can participate and communicate appropriately for each situation.

Hearing Impaired Patients. Be sensitive to the potential for patients to have hearing impairment. Do not assume that all people with hearing impairment can read lips or understand American Sign Language (ASL); also do not assume that a hearing aid returns the patient's hearing to normal. Do not assume that hearing impaired patients have diminished intellectual abilities.

Many pharmacists are quite skilled in ASL, used by the Deaf in the United States and English-speaking Canadians, or they can finger-spell words using the ASL alphabet. ASL courses and seminars are widely available. Regardless of the level of special skills obtained, communicate as clearly as possible with hearing impaired patients. Verbalize slowly and distinctly; minimize background noise. Face patients who can read laps and avoid turning away from the patient during the conversation. Written communication may be necessary for two-way communication.

Critically Ill Patients.   The intensive care unit is a highly depersonalizing environment. Patients have little privacy or sense of control. Families and friends may feel overwhelmed. Patients are surrounded by high-tech equipment and may be sleep deprived; drowsy from pain medication; or uncomfortable from procedures, tests, or surgery. This environment makes it difficult to relate to the patient as a person. Nevertheless, it is important to communicate directly with the patient. Speak to the patient when entering or leaving the patient's room, even if the patient appears unresponsive. Never assume that the patient cannot hear or comprehend what is said in his or her presence. Make eye contact with the patient, even if it means getting very close to the patient's face. Endotracheal intubation renders patients mute but do not assume that intubated patients cannot communicate. Intubated patients can respond to yes/no questions by blinking their eyes or raising an arm. Some intubated patients can express themselves in writing if the paper is positioned for them or use point and spell boards. Acknowledge and communicate directly with the patient's family and friends, who may be very anxious or frustrated.

Chronically Ill Patients.   Chronically ill patients present unique communication challenges. Chronically ill patients may be sophisticated and/or demanding health care consumers. Some chronically ill patients know more about the management of their disease than many health care professionals; this situation may be threatening for the pharmacist. Some chronically ill patients may be completely disillusioned by repeated unsatisfactory interactions with the health care system and may be bitter, cynical, and difficult to engage in conversation.

Chronically ill patients deserve the same amount of information and attention as all other patients. Assess the needs of each patient and be flexible enough to communicate on an appropriate level. Discussing sophisticated therapeutic regimens may be a pleasure with pleasant and well-informed patients but extremely difficult with bitter, cynical patients. Chronically ill patients must learn to live with their disease; this may take years and may never be fully accomplished.

Terminally Ill Patients.   Terminally ill patients may be sophisticated and/or demanding health care consumers as well; they also may be bitter, cynical, and difficult to engage in conversation. Terminally ill patients often take complicated drug regimens requiring detailed instruction and monitoring. Many terminally ill patients and their families have to deal with the stigma of frequent prescriptions for high-dose narcotics.

Treat terminally ill patients with respect and work with them to achieve optimal therapeutic efficacy within the complexities of their illnesses and the health care environment. Terminally ill patients may need help dealing with complex insurance paperwork and complex medication regimens. Terminally ill patients need close monitoring and reassurance about their medication regimens. Some terminally ill patients require large and frequent doses of narcotics; work with the patient and their family to legitimize the use of these medications and minimize the hassles associated with obtaining narcotics.

Hard-to-Reach Patients.   Hard-to-reach patients include those of low socioeconomic status, minorities, and illiterate persons.[10] Communicating with these patients may be difficult. Patients of low socioeconomic status have few resources to deal with health care issues. They may have little knowledge about health care in general and their own health in particular and may have different coping mechanisms and expectations. They may not have the economic or social resources to participate in preventive health care or manage acute or chronic illness. Pharmacists must be sensitive to these issues.

Look beyond these issues and communicate clearly and directly with each patient as an individual, regardless of the patient's status. Hard-to-reach patients deserve as much respect, time, and information as do all other patients and should not be glossed over and dismissed because of their socioeconomic status, ethnic origin, or illiteracy. The health care needs of hard-to-reach patients often are greater than those of other patients; be sensitive to their needs. Help illiterate patients organize complex medication regimens by using different-sized bottles for each medication or color-coding the labels. Calendars with dosages of unit-of-use medication stapled to the appropriate date may help illiterate patients adhere to complex medication regimens. Other medication-delivery devices may help patients keep track of their doses.

Be sensitive to the cost of medications and the ability of the patient to pay for the medication. Low-income elderly patients in particular may be too embarrassed to ask about the cost of medications and may accept expensive medications they cannot afford. Less expensive, therapeutically acceptable alternative medications usually are available. Some pharmaceutical companies have patient assistance programs that provide select medications free of charge to individuals without third-party prescription coverage and who meet specific income requirements.

Antagonistic Patients.   Antagonistic patients do not want to be bothered with medication histories, interviews, or other pharmacist-patient interactions. The natural response to these patients is to leave them alone and avoid them if possible. However, these patients deserve as much attention as other patients and may need more attention from the pharmacist because their behavior alienates them from other health care professionals. The best ways to deal with such patients are to be as professional and direct as possible and limit the length of the interaction to as short a period as possible. These patients may be frightened or simply fed up with the entire health care system; therefore clarification of the purpose of and reasons for the interaction and the ways in which the information obtained from the interaction are used may be helpful. Most patients have a great deal of respect for pharmacists and cooperate if the need for the interaction is clearly defined and they perceive that they are treated with respect.

Noncommunicative and Overly Communicative Patients.   Noncommunicative and overly communicative patients present special challenges. Noncommunicative patients never volunteer information or express much interest in anything anyone has to say. These patients answer all questions with unenthusiastic yes/no responses. To facilitate communication, get the patient talking about any topic and then ask simple, open-ended questions that will provide at least some of the information being sought during the interaction. For example, patients unwilling to identify the medications they are currently taking may open up and start discussing their medication if asked to describe their satisfaction with past medication. Sometimes no communication method works and the communication remains one way. However, most patients can be drawn out and encouraged to engage in effective two-way communication.

Overly communicative patients digress when asked even simple direct questions. Pharmacists eventually obtain the information being sought, but only after investing a lot of time in the interview. The best way to deal with this type of patient is to take firm control of the conversation from the start and redirect the patient when he or she wanders off the subject. The patient may have to be allowed to wander a little before being gently but firmly interrupted and redirected. For example, a patient may be eager to discuss a pet dog's medical problems. The pharmacist may need to give the patient a few moments to talk about these issues before redirecting the patient back to the focus of the interview.

COMMUNICATING WITH HEALTH CARE PROFESSIONALS

Effective communication between pharmacists and physicians, nurses, and other pharmacists is essential. Poor communication not only leads to frustration and lack of respect among professions but also may compromise patient care if important information is misunderstood, ineffectively conveyed, or left out.

Pharmacist-Physician Communication. Pharmacists and physicians often have trouble communicating with one another. Both professionals are extremely busy; communication usually takes place when neither party has much time to converse. Many pharmacists are intimidated by physicians (Figure 2-3). Pharmacists must be comfortable with their role on the health care team and confident in their unique knowledge and contributions to patient care.

Be prepared with specific questions or facts and recommendations when initiating a patient care–related conversation with physicians. Make sure other resources cannot answer the question. Stay within the pharmacist's area of expertise. Choose the right time and place for the conversation. Never interrupt a physician-patient interaction, except for life-threatening situations. Follow the chain of command. Do not go to an attending physician when the question or recommendation is more appropriate for a less senior member of the medical team. Do not interrupt teaching rounds with trivial questions and observations better communicated one-to-one with individual physicians. Do not engage physicians in lengthy social small talk.

If the physician initiates the conversation, listen carefully, assess the information or question, and ask for additional information until the question is clear and specific. Physician-initiated questions often are vague and general. Clarify the question and obtain appropriate patient-related data. For example, a physician may ask if a serum digoxin concentration of 0.8 µg/L is okay. Given that the usual therapeutic range is 0.8 to 2 µg/L, the initial instinct is to verify that a concentration of 0.8 µg/L is okay. However, the question should not be answered until the pharmacist finds out when the blood sample was obtained, when drug therapy was initiated, why the drug was prescribed, the clinical status of the patient, and the goal of therapy.

Pharmacist-Nurse Communication. Pharmacists and nurses often have trouble communicating with one another. Pharmacists and nurses are extremely busy; communication often occurs when neither party has much time to spend conversing. Unfortunately, most pharmacist-nurse communication takes place because of drug distribution errors; much of the tension between the two professions is based on these interactions. Nurses are pressed to obtain and administer medication, and pharmacists are frustrated because nonstat requests often are presented as emergencies (e.g., stat docusate sodium). The pharmacist and the nurse end up in a tug-of-war over work priorities, which can lead to lack of respect and poor communication on

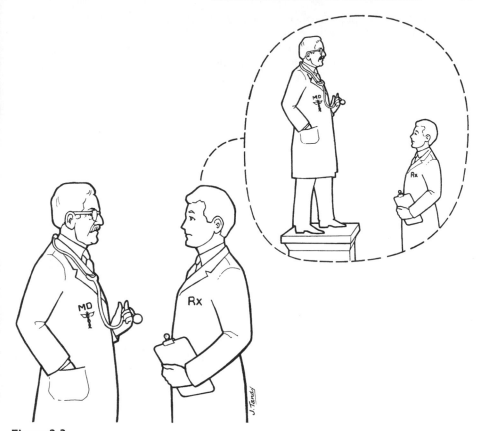

Figure 2-3
Pharmacist-Physician Communication.
Pharmacists often have difficulty communicating with physicians because they feel intimidated.

the part of both professionals. Pharmacists and nurses must treat one another with respect; both professionals must realize that they share the same goal (e.g., optimal patient care) and are on the same patient care team. Communication should be clear, to the point, and timely.

An added barrier to effective pharmacist-nurse communication is the use of the telephone as the primary means of communication. It is easy to be rude, either intentionally or unintentionally. Feelings get hurt and reputations lost when tempers flare during less-than-optimal telephone interactions.

Pharmacist-Pharmacist Communication.   Patient care may be less than optimal because of communication difficulties between pharmacists. For example, pharmacists on consult services such as pharmacokinetics or infectious disease may not have access to recent uncharted patient information or be privy to in-depth discussions during team rounds. Pharmacists on the patient care team need to update consulting pharmacists frequently. Consulting pharmacists should be aware that the primary team may have more information than that documented in the patient record; they should not make recommendations in isolation.

Inpatient patient-focused care takes place 24 hours a day, 7 days a week. Continuity between shifts requires clear communication of patient information, plans for the patient, and other patient issues. A common communication system is the exchange of patient information during sign-out rounds or the discussion of patient-specific issues and the passing on of patient monitoring forms and other types of written documentation between the pharmacists leaving the service and those assuming responsibility for the patient.

Community pharmacists and institutional pharmacists rarely share patient-related information. Although patients and other members of the health care team potentially benefit by knowing details regarding patient's medications and status before hospitalization and upon discharge, the fragmented nature of traditional health care delivery systems makes this type of communication nearly impossible. Unified health care delivery systems may allow for more information to be communicated among pharmacists as patients move between ambulatory and acute care environments.

ADDITIONAL COMMUNICATION SKILLS

TEACHING

Many nonfaculty pharmacists teach in a variety of settings, including one-on-one individualized patient teaching, small group patient support groups, and seminars and lectures for pharmacy and other health care students. Community, institutional, and industry pharmacists may have a variety of classroom teaching responsibilities at nearby colleges of pharmacy, nursing, or medicine (e.g., lectures, recitations, laboratories). Although many pharmacists teach, most have little formal training.

A teacher must be well organized and knowledgeable about the subject being taught and must be an excellent communicator. Communication is enhanced by having good organizational skills. The structure of the session and material should be obvious without the use of written handouts. Introduce topics and summarize periodically. Interact with the audience during the teaching session to determine the depth of the participant's understanding and change or redirect the focus of the lecture or discussion to meet the needs of the audience. Direct questioning and assessment of responses are easy ways to determine whether the students and participant understand the material; however, these methods are less effective in large classroom settings. Feedback in formal classroom settings comes primarily from nonverbal behavior. Participants who understand and comprehend the material are quiet, focused, and obviously thinking. Participants who are confused or do not understand the material being presented shift uneasily in their seat, converse with those around them, engage in other activities (e.g., reading a newspaper), or sleep.

Pharmacy clerkships typically consist of one-on-one or small group teaching sessions. The student and teacher review individual patient cases and discuss the pathophysiologic and therapeutic issues. Many students are intimidated by the highly individualized nature of this type of one-on-one teaching. Put the student at ease while controlling the educational aspect of the interactions. Students also may feel intimidated or threatened by a constant barrage of seemingly unrelated questions. An effective communication tool during these types of teaching sessions is the circular questioning technique. This technique involves guiding the student through a series of related, basic questions that eventually lead the student to discover the correct answer to a previously asked question. Then ask a series of increasingly difficult questions, allowing the student to reinforce the material already learned while applying and learning new information. Frequent verbal summaries and constructive feedback are essential teaching tools.

PLATFORM AND POSTER PRESENTATIONS

Platform Presentations. Many pharmacists make platform presentations at local, state, and national professional meetings. However, most pharmacists have little experience with these types of presentations. Audiences range from less than a dozen people to several hundred and include pharmacists as well as other health care professionals. Many pharmacists are stressed by public speaking. Although the degree of stress felt by the speaker depends on the individual and the specific situation, some degree of stress is perfectly natural. Stress is reduced through experience and thorough preparation. However, many experienced speakers still admit to being nervous before and during presentations. Some speakers find they can reduce stress by acknowledging the anxiety rather then denying their feelings. The nervous energy generated by stress can be directed into enthusiasm for the topic and increased energy during the presentation.

Reduce stress by selecting an appropriate topic. Speaking about a familiar topic is much easier than speaking about a less familiar topic. Be well informed and well prepared. Minimize stress by considering the audience and targeting the level of information to the audience's background. This helps create interest on the part of the audience, which in turn provides positive feedback to the speaker. Learn how to operate all the audiovisual equipment before starting the presentation. Reduce the stress of answering audience questions by anticipating and preparing answers to likely questions.

Use appropriate audiovisual materials. A good visual image presents information more vividly and accurately than lengthy verbal descriptions. For example, a videotape of a patient having a grand mal seizure provides visual images that cannot be obtained from oral descriptions. Create well-designed slides (Box 2-4), transparencies (Box 2-5) and audio tapes. Currently available computer programs enable creation of sophisticated images and integration of multiple audiovisual formats. Design visual images to enhance rather than replace orally presented information. Design the images so that all members of the audiences can see the images and read all the information presented.

BOX 2-4

Slide Design*

> Use simple font styles.
> Limit each slide to one idea, figure, or table.
> Use a horizontal rather than a vertical format.
> Use no more than 5 or 6 lines per slide.
> Use a 2-to-3 horizontal/vertical ratio for each slide.
> Use colors to highlight information, but do not use more than 2 or 3 colors.
> Use bright, clear colors; avoid pastels and neon colors.
> Use simple tables and graphs.

*Electronic slides and 35-mm slides.

BOX 2-5

Transparency Design

Use simple font styles.
Use letters large enough to be read from a distance.
Limit each transparency to one idea, figure, or table.
Use no more than 5 or 6 words per line.
Use no more than 5 or 6 lines per transparency.

Poster Presentations.   The poster presentation is a unique communication format in which the information is displayed rather than orally presented. Although most poster sessions require the author to be available to answer questions and discuss the information presented, the visual image of the poster is what grabs the attention of passersby and draws them in for more detailed perusal. Posters that attract the most attention have clear, descriptive titles and a colorful, neat, and professional appearance.

The allocated space dictates the amount of information presented in the poster. The amount of space allocated for each poster varies from meeting to meeting; requirements and limitations are communicated to the presenter when the poster is accepted for presentation. Most posters include a descriptive title, names of the individuals presenting the data, abstract, introduction, background information, study design, data, results, and conclusions. Printed material should be readable from several feet away. Brightly colored backgrounds enhance the visual presentation. Visual aids such as tables, graphs, charts, and photographs communicate information more effectively than multiple pages of text.

MEDIA INTERVIEWS

Pharmacists may be called by the media to provide background information regarding therapeutic issues such as the marketing of an important new drug, a widely publicized drug-related problem, or the withdrawal of a drug from the market. Media interviews can be interesting and rewarding experiences that provide a positive and effective form of communication between pharmacists and the public. However, pharmacists need to remember that journalists are not health care professionals and may misunderstand or use information out of context. Be cognizant of the very short deadlines most journalists have to meet; journalists may need information for a news report scheduled to air in just a few hours. Journalists can be quite aggressive. A media expert noted, "If you don't learn to use the media to your advantage, you will be used by it."[11]

Most media contact is by telephone. Determine the contact's name, telephone number or e-mail address, organization, position, how the information is going to be used, and the exact issue of interest. Do not answer any questions, divulge any information, or provide any opinions without knowing this information. Some members of the less-than-reputable media do not offer this information unless specifically prompted. Members of the legitimate media understand the importance of this information and readily disclose these facts.

Prepare to speak with a journalist by reviewing the subject to be discussed. Anticipate related or tangential issues and be prepared to elaborate on the topic and to explain technical terminology and concepts in lay language. Speak with other individuals who have been interviewed by the reporter or read articles published by the journalist to get a feel for the person's style. After the interview, ensure that the information obtained by the journalist is accurate. No one wants to be misquoted or quoted out of context. Be available for clarification by telephone, fax, or e-mail. Some print-format publishers ask sources to review and verify the information before publication.

MANUSCRIPTS

Original research reports, case studies, review articles, editorials, and letters to the editor are important communication tools among health care professionals worldwide. Publishing these types of articles in the print media is an important but challenging activity. Successful publication requires excellent writing skills as well as careful planning and execution of the plan.

One of the most important decisions made when attempting to publish a manuscript is selecting the appropriate journal. Match the focus and type of manuscript with the focus and audience of the journal. For example, editors of the *Journal of Infectious Diseases* are not interested in publishing a manuscript about a drug used to treat gastrointestinal bleeding. Other common mistakes include trying to publish information already well documented in the literature, submitting a poorly designed and/or executed study, submitting a poorly written manuscript, and not following journal-specific guidelines. Well-written manuscripts that meet the needs of the journal's audience will be published.

SELF-ASSESSMENT QUESTIONS

1. Active listening consists of which of the following tasks?
   a. Focusing on what the other person says
   b. Assessing the way the other person communicates
   c. Conveying an open, relaxed, and unhurried attitude
   d. All of the above
   e. None of the above

2. To convey interest and attentiveness, the pharmacist should do which of the following?
   a. Avoid eye contact.
   b. Stand or sit at eye level or lower.
   c. Stand or sit as close to the person as possible.
   d. Ignore the other person's body language.
   e. Take copious notes during the interview.

3. Barriers to verbal communication are minimized in which of the following settings?
   a. The interview takes place through a window with security bars.
   b. The interview takes place in front of three of the patient's hospital roommates.
   c. The interview is conducted over the telephone.
   d. The patient is interviewed in a private consultation office.
   e. The patient is interviewed through a drive-in window.

4. Which one of the following is *not* an important consideration when writing medical record notes?
   a. Use black ink.
   b. Write clearly and legibly.
   c. Title the note with a specific heading.
   d. Document the facts and avoiding unsubstantiated judgments.
   e. Begin the note on an unused page.

5. When is addressing a patient by the first name appropriate?
   a. When a patient is disoriented
   b. When meeting a patient for the first time
   c. When trying to placate a patient
   d. When a patient is much older than the pharmacist
   e. When a patient is much younger than the pharmacist

6. What kind of questions should be asked early in a patient interview?
   a. Long, complex questions
   b. Questions that can be answered "yes" or "no"
   c. Open-ended questions
   d. Leading questions
   e. Multiple questions

7. Which of the following may make an embarrassing situation worse?
   a. Being aware of potentially embarrassing situations
   b. Being sensitive to clues that the patient is embarrassed
   c. Using humor to relieve the tension
   d. Discussing the issue in a scientifically appropriate manner
   e. Communicating with the patient in privacy

8. The best way to deal with antagonistic patients is to do which of the following?
   a. Avoid them.
   b. Suggest less expensive alternative medications.
   c. Talk with their legal guardians.
   d. Speak slowly and distinctly.
   e. Limit the length of each interaction.

9. The best way to deal with physically challenged patients is to do which of the following?
   a. Treat them like any other patient.
   b. Avoid making eye contact.
   c. Stare at them.
   d. Ignore them.
   e. Physically assist them without asking permission.

10. Stress associated with platform presentations can be reduced by doing which of the following?
    a. Targeting the material for the specific audience
    b. Acknowledging the presentation as a stressful situation
    c. Anticipating and preparing for audience questions
    d. All of the above
    e. None of the above

References

1. How should patients be addressed? AORN 31:1142-1144, 1146, 1148, 1980.
2. Ranelli PL, Svarstadt BL, Boh L: Factors affecting outcomes of medication-history interviewing by pharmacy students, Am J Hosp Pharm 46:267-281, 1989.
3. Zakus GE et al: Teaching interviewing for pediatrics, J Med Ed 51:325-331, 1976.
4. Ivey M, Tso Y, Stamm K: Communication techniques for patient instruction, Am J Hosp Pharm 32:828-831, 1975.
5. Shaughnessy AF: Patients' understanding of selected pharmacy terms, Am Pharm NS28(10):38-42, 1988.

6. Oliver CH: Communication awareness: Rx for embarrassing situations, *Am Pharm* NS22(10):21-23, 1982.
7. Galizia VJ, Sause RB: Communicating with the geriatric patient, *Am Pharm* NS22(10):35-36, 1982.
8. Portnoy E: Enhancing communication with elderly patients, *Am Pharm* NS25(8):50-55, 1985.
9. Eigen BN: Improving communication with the physically disabled, *Am Pharm* NS22(10):37-40, 1982.
10. Freimuth VS, Mettger W: Is there a hard-to-reach audience? *Pub Health Rep* 105:232-238, 1990.
11. Experts offer advice on dealing with the media, *Mich Med* 89:19-20, 1990.

Taking Medication Histories

3

CHAPTER

Learning Objectives

- State the advantages and disadvantages of interviewing patients before and after review of patient information.
- Identify relevant information obtained from observing the patient's appearance and environment.
- List the categories of data obtained during a medication history interview.
- Describe the type of information included in each category of data obtained during a medication history interview.
- Express a patient's smoking history in terms of pack-years.
- Differentiate between an allergy and an adverse drug reaction.
- State how to assess patient compliance with prescribed or recommended medication regimens.
- Identify types of questions to avoid when interviewing patients.
- Identify types of patients who are difficult to interview. Describe the most effective ways to interview these types of patients.
- Discuss the advantages and disadvantages of documenting the patient medication history using a standardized form, the SOAP format, and the freestyle format.

Historically, pharmacists relied on physicians, nurses, and other health care professionals to obtain and document information regarding medications taken by patients. Many medications at the turn of the century were relatively ineffective and had few risks, so most health care professionals had little interest in obtaining detailed medication histories. Pharmacists had limited direct patient care responsibility and did not need firsthand knowledge of patient medication use.

Today, medication histories obtained by nonpharmacists are generally sketchy and lack important information regarding medication allergies and sensitivities, prescription and nonprescription medication use, alternative remedies, and reliability in taking scheduled doses.[1,2] Recognition of the increasing availability of potent prescription and nonprescription medications and the increasingly fragmented health care system has renewed interest in the need for pharmacist-acquired and pharmacist-documented medication histories.

The medication history is the foundation for planning optimal patient-specific medication regimens. The medication history is the starting point for generating hypotheses regarding the patient's understanding of the role of medications in the treatment of disease; the patient's ability to comply with the medication regimen; the medication's effectiveness; and the patient's experiences with side effects, allergies, and adverse drug reactions.

Pharmacists have a unique combination of drug-related expertise and experience; patients trust and respect pharmacists. Although other health care professionals interview patients regarding their use of medications, no other health care professional has the pharmacist's depth and scope of knowledge regarding medications. Therefore it is important that pharmacists obtain and document patient medication histories and communicate this information to the rest of the health care team.

Obtaining medication histories is not just a matter of common sense and experience. Although interviewing is a creative process that is somewhat difficult to define, successful interviewing requires excellent patient-oriented process skills (Box 3-1) and communication process skills (Box 3-2); pharmacists must be aware of and avoid common hindering behaviors (Box 3-3).[3-5]

PREPARATION FOR THE INTERVIEW

There are two distinctly different approaches to preparing for a patient interview. One approach is to review all that is known about the patient's medical condition and medications and then target the interview to specific issues identified during the review. This approach is commonly used when patients are admitted to acute care or long-term care institutions where physicians and nurses have already documented at least some patient information. The advantages of this approach are that the pharmacist has some knowledge of the patient before the interview and can prepare to explore and address specific issues; the pharmacist may feel more comfortable having this knowledge before interacting with the patient. The disadvantage of this approach is that important information may be overlooked if the pharmacist becomes too focused or unduly influenced by previously obtained information.

The other approach is to interview the patient before reviewing any previously documented patient information. Community-based pharmacists rarely have access to information about patients and must be able to conduct effective interviews without knowing the patients or their histories. The advantage of this approach is that the pharmacist is completely unbiased about each patient and the patient's history, thus allowing the exploration of all aspects of the medication history with equal intensity. The disadvantage of this approach is that it can be an intimidating and time-consuming process for the inexperienced interviewer.

OBSERVATION OF THE PATIENT AND THE PATIENT'S ENVIRONMENT

Close observation of the patient and the patient's immediate surroundings provides important information regarding the patient's state of health, economic status, compliance with specific dietary recommendations, and social support system.[6] These data help the pharmacist select and monitor the outcomes of specific medication regimens. For example, drugs used to manage hypertension may appear ineffective if the patient refuses to comply with salt or other dietary restrictions. Patients may choose to pay the rent rather than buy expensive medications. Patients may not understand complex medication regimens or may not be able to prepare and admin-

BOX 3-1

Patient-Oriented Process Skills

1. Knock on the door and request permission to enter the room of the institutionalized patient.
2. Introduce yourself.
3. Try to achieve privacy.
4. Make sure the patient is comfortable.
5. Communicate at eye level or lower.
6. Remove distractions (loud television and radio, relatives, and friends).
7. Clarify the purpose of the interview.
8. Obtain the patient's permission for the interview.
9. Verify the patient's name and correct pronunciation.
10. Address the patient by the appropriate title.
11. Maintain eye contact with the patient.

From Zakus GE et al: J Med Ed 51:325-331, 1976; Lipkin M Jr, Quill TE, Napodano RJ: Ann Intern Med 100:277-284, 1984; and Preven DW et al: J Med Ed 61:842-844, 1986.

BOX 3-2

Communication Skills

1. Provide clear instructions regarding the structure of the interview and expectations for the patient.
2. Use a balance of open-ended and closed-ended questions.
3. Use vocabulary geared to the patient.
4. Use nonbiased questions.
5. Give the patient time to respond.
6. Interrupt or redirect as necessary but do not interrupt when the patient is on track.
7. Listen to the patient; do not cut off the patient.
8. Discuss one topic at a time.
9. Move from general to specific topics.
10. Pursue unclear questions until they are clarified.
11. Ask simple questions.
12. Identify and recognize patient feelings. Verbally acknowledge appropriate or hostile feelings.
13. Give feedback to the patient. Ask, "Is this what you mean?"
14. Obtain feedback from the patient.
15. Attend to patient cues (posture, tone of voice, affect).
16. Invite the patient to ask questions.
17. Answer patient questions.
18. Use transitional statements and summarization.
19. Close the interview.

From Zakus GE et al: J Med Ed 51:325-331, 1976; Lipkin M Jr, Quill TE, Napodano RJ: Ann Intern Med 100:277-284, 1984; and Preven DW et al: J Med Ed 61:842-844, 1986.

BOX 3-3

Hindering Behaviors

Using technical language and medical jargon
Frequently interrupting the patient
Asking leading questions
Allowing frequent external interruptions (phone calls, beepers)
Expressing bias and personal prejudices
Maintaining a closed posture
Reading notes and charts during the interview
Projecting a superior or threatening posture
Avoiding eye contact with the patient
Engaging in sarcasm
Making derogatory statements about other health care professionals
Ignoring emotion displayed by the patient
Speaking too quickly or too slowly or mumbling
Asking multiple questions
Asking rapid-fire questions
Perpetuating cultural barriers

From Zakus GE et al: J Med Ed 51:325-331, 1976; Lipkin M Jr, Quill TE, Napodano RJ: Ann Intern Med 100:277-284, 1984; and Preven DW et al: J Med Ed 61:842-844, 1986.

ister nonoral dosage formulations (e.g., subcutaneous medications, inhaled medications, suppositories).

A patient's general well-being and socioeconomic class can be judged by how the patient is dressed. An unkempt appearance or sloppy dress may indicate that the patient is too ill to pay attention to these details. Other clues to the patient's lifestyle and sense of well-being include make-up, hairstyle, location and number of body piercings, hearing aids, and watches with large numbers or Braille faces. The amount, quality, and type of jewelry provide some information about a patient's socioeconomic status.

Carefully observe the patient for the type, amount, pattern of wear, degree of tidiness, and general fit of clothing. Worn, dated clothing suggests that the patient may have difficulty paying for prescribed therapies. Patterns of wear on shoes and shirt-sleeves may suggest physical impairment from stroke or other trauma. Long sleeves and broad-brimmed hats inappropriate to the season suggest photosensitivity or an attempt to hide track marks or scars from suicide attempts, trauma, or surgery. Shoes with toes and other areas cut out suggest a history of gout or other joint disease. Oversized clothing may indicate recent weight loss; too-tight clothing may indicate recent weight gain. Note whether belts are buckled at usual wear spots or if the patient has let the belt out or tightened it up. Loose-fitting house slippers or untied sneakers may indicate recent lower extremity edema. A predominance of snaps, zippers, and Velcro-type fastenings may indicate loss of manual dexterity. A patient with hypothyroidism may dress too warmly; a patient with hyperthyroidism may dress too coolly. Do not, however, read too much into these observations; evaluate these observations in context with the rest of the data obtained during the patient interview.

Carefully observe an institutionalized patient's room. Flowers, plants, get-well cards, and children's drawings indicate that the patient has family and friends who are aware of the patient's illness and are providing social support. Books, newspapers, and magazines indicate that the patient is literate and provide clues about the patient's outside interests. Reading material, crossword puzzles, and crafts such as knitting also indicate that the patient feels well enough to engage in these activities.

The presence of food in a patient's room has several potential meanings. Food gift baskets indicate social support but may indicate potential problems for patients on restricted diets. Food left from prior meals may indicate that the patient is not hungry, has missed a meal while at a test or procedure, or dislikes the institutional food; many drugs suppress the appetite and contribute to anorexia. Food from home may indicate that the patient dislikes the institutional food or that family and friends are trying to supply special foods and treats to entice a patient to eat. Look for extra or forbidden food in the rooms of patients with diabetes, heavily salted snack foods in the rooms of patients on salt-restricted diets, and soft drinks or water in the rooms of patients who are fluid restricted. Dietary indiscretions may be primary or contributing factors in failure of prescribed therapeutic regimens.

DATA TO BE OBTAINED

Data obtained during the medication history interview include demographic information, dietary information, social habits, current and past prescription and non-prescription medications and alternative remedies, allergies, adverse drug reactions, and adherence with prescribed or recommended medication regimens (Box 3-4). The data obtained should be as complete and descriptive as possible.

DEMOGRAPHIC INFORMATION

Demographic information includes the patient's age, height, weight, race and ethnic origin, education, occupation, and lifestyle. Lifestyle information includes the patient's housing situation (e.g., boarding house, private home, apartment, shelter, living on the street), people living with the patient (e.g., spouse, young children, elderly relatives, extended family), and the patient's type of work and work schedule, if applicable (i.e., day shift, night shift, rotating shift schedules, part-time, full-time). All of these factors influence decisions regarding the selection of prescription and nonprescription medication, the dosage of the medication, and the therapeutic regimen. For example, patients who work with machinery may choose not to take medications that make them drowsy, sluggish, or shaky. Patients with restricted work breaks may be reluctant to take diuretic medications. Patients who live in shelters may not have access to refrigeration. Patients hesitant to give themselves injections may be unwilling to take these types of medications unless someone is available to help them.

DIETARY INFORMATION

Dietary information includes the type of diet and dietary restrictions (if any), supplements, and stimulants. For example, patients with diabetes may follow the American Diabetic Association (ADA) dietary guidelines; other patients may be on recommended or self-imposed low-fat, low-sodium, low-calorie, low-fiber, or high-fiber diets. Some drug therapies may appear ineffective if the patient is noncompliant with recommended dietary restrictions (e.g., patients with congestive heart failure may not comply with salt-restricted diets). Patients may self-medicate with nonprescription

BOX 3-4

Data to Be Obtained from a Medication History Interview

DEMOGRAPHIC INFORMATION
Age
Height and weight
Race and ethnic origin
Residence
Education
Occupation

DIETARY INFORMATION
Dietary restrictions
Dietary supplements
Dietary stimulants
Dietary suppressants

SOCIAL HABITS
Tobacco
Alcohol
Illicit drugs

CURRENT PRESCRIPTION MEDICATIONS
Name and description
Dosage
Dosing schedule (prescribed and actual)
Indications
Date medication started
Outcome of therapy

PAST PRESCRIPTION MEDICATIONS
Name and description
Dosage
Dosing schedule (prescribed and actual)
Indication
Date medication started
Date medication stopped
Reason for stopping the medication
Outcome of therapy

CURRENT NONPRESCRIPTION MEDICATIONS
Name and description
Dosage
Dosing schedule (recommended and actual)
Indication
Date medication started
Outcome of therapy

PAST NONPRESCRIPTION MEDICATIONS
Name and description
Dosage

Continued

BOX 3-4

Data to Be Obtained from a Medication History Interview—cont'd

PAST NONPRESCRIPTION MEDICATIONS—cont'd
Dosing schedule (recommended and actual)
Indication
Date medication started
Date medication stopped
Reason for stopping the medication
Outcome of therapy

CURRENT AND PAST ALTERNATIVE REMEDIES
Name and description
Dosage
Dosing schedule
Indication
Date remedy started
Date remedy stopped (if applicable)
Reason for stopping the medication (if applicable)
Outcome of therapy

ALLERGIES
Name and description of causative agent
Dosage
Date of reaction
Description of reaction
How the reaction was treated

ADVERSE DRUG REACTIONS
Name and description
Dosage
Date of reaction
Description of reaction
How the reaction was treated

COMPLIANCE

dietary supplements, stimulants, or suppressants that interact adversely with prescribed medications and treatment regimens.

SOCIAL HABITS
Social habits include the use of tobacco, alcohol, and illicit drugs. Document the duration of use, amount of each agent consumed, frequency of use, and reasons for use of each agent without being judgmental. Determine the type, quantity, pattern, and duration of alcohol use. To assess tobacco use, note the age at which the patient first started smoking tobacco and when (if applicable) the patient quit smoking. Because the effects of smoking on drug metabolism may be clinically important for weeks to months after the patient has stopped smoking, note approximately when the patient stopped smoking. Acute care pharmacists should be especially sensitive

to these issues; patients often quit smoking just before hospitalization and may consider themselves nonsmokers when asked about their smoking habits.

Tobacco smoking is quantified in terms of packs per day and expressed in pack-years (e.g., 2 packs per day for 5 years; 10 pack-years). One pack-year is equivalent to smoking 1 pack of cigarettes daily for 1 year. A 10 pack-year tobacco history is equivalent to smoking half a pack per day for 20 years, one pack per day for 10 years, or two packs per day for 5 years.

Illicit drug use may be difficult to ascertain. Obtain this information in a professional, nonthreatening, nonjudgmental manner. Do not try to guess which patients are more or less likely to use these agents but probe for this information with every patient. Surprisingly, patients may be more comfortable revealing this type of information to pharmacists than to other health care professionals, including physicians. Patients generally do not understand the term *illicit;* the best approach is to ask about the use of so-called street drugs and give an example or two such as marijuana, crack cocaine, and heroin. Document the amount of each agent consumed; the frequency, pattern, and duration of use; and the reasons for use of each agent.

CURRENT PRESCRIPTION MEDICATIONS

Obtain a complete description of current prescription medications from the patient, including the name and dosage of the drug, dosing schedule (prescribed and actual), duration of therapy, reason the patient is taking the medication, and outcome of therapy. Knowledge of current prescription medications allows the pharmacist to evaluate the efficacy and safety of prescribed regimens.

Patients may not be able to remember the names of all their medications. If this is the case, obtain a detailed description of each medication, including the dosage form (e.g., tablet, capsule, liquid, topical); size, shape, and color of the dosage form; and any words, letters, and numbers on the dosage form that the patient can remember. If the patient cannot remember the dosage of the drug, the pharmacist may be able to identify the drug and/or dosage from other details the patient provides. However, clearly document the patient's description and note that the medication might be a specific product. For example, a patient may note taking a purple capsule with three yellow rings on the capsule for indigestion. Although this is likely Nexium (esomeprazole) 40 mg, document the patient's description and note that the description is consistent with Nexium 40 mg.

Obtain the prescribed dosing schedule (e.g., four times a day, two times a day, once a day) and note the routine times the patient takes each dose. If a discrepancy between the prescribed dosing schedule and the schedule the patient uses is apparent (e.g., the patient is supposed to take the medication four times a day but takes it two times a day), note the discrepancy and try to determine the reason the patient uses the drug differently from how it is prescribed. Patients sometimes change dosing schedules to fit their work schedules and lifestyles or to conserve medication to reduce the expenses of chronic medications.

Many prescription medications are taken "as needed" (PRN); as a result, ascertaining the amount of prescription medication used by the patient may be difficult. However, quantification is important; do not accept imprecise descriptive terms. For example, the term *occasional* may mean anything from one dose of the medication every few months to one or more doses per day. One approach to quantifying the amount of medication actually consumed by the patient is to inquire how often the patient has to obtain a new supply of the medication. This information provides an indirect assessment of the amount of medication the patient actually takes over average periods of time.

Try to determine exactly when the patient started taking the prescription medication and the reason the patient gives for taking the medication. Exact dates are important in determining whether an adverse or allergic reaction is a result of a specific medication and whether the prescribed medications are effectively treating or controlling a specific condition. For example, a patient with elevated blood pressure may claim to be compliant with his or her blood pressure medication. The decision to continue or discontinue the medication depends on when the patient started the current regimen. The regimen would continue unchanged if the patient had just started the medication last week but would need to be changed if the patient had been taking the medication for 2 months. Some patients may not know the specific reason they are taking their medications because they misunderstand the reason it has been prescribed. Document the reasons the patient gives for taking the medication and clarify any discrepancies regarding usual uses of medications with the prescriber, not the patient.

PAST PRESCRIPTION MEDICATIONS
Obtain as much information about past prescription medications as possible, including name and description, dosage, prescribed and actual dosing schedule, dates and duration of therapy, reason for taking the medication, and outcome. Knowledge of past prescriptions helps the pharmacist understand the medications used, either successfully or unsuccessfully, to treat current and past medical problems; this knowledge guides recommendations regarding new medication regimens. Patients are unlikely to remember all these details for past medications. Document the details the patient can remember; avoid excessive "grilling" of the patient.

Document any other information the patient provides about the past medications as well as the reason the patient stopped taking the medication. Medication regimens may be short and well defined, as with antibiotic therapy, or multiple medications may be tried over a prolonged period in an effort to find an effective medication with an acceptable side effect profile.

CURRENT NONPRESCRIPTION MEDICATIONS
Obtain a complete description of current nonprescription medications from the patient. Document the name and dosage of the drug, recommended and actual dosing schedule, dates and duration of therapy, reason the patient is taking the medication, and outcome of therapy. Knowledge of current nonprescription medications allows the pharmacist to determine whether drug interactions may occur between prescribed and self-administered medications, whether the patient is self-medicating to relieve an adverse drug reaction from a prescribed medication or in an attempt to obtain better relief from symptoms than that provided with the prescribed regimen, and whether a nonprescription medication is the cause of a patient's complaint or is exacerbating a concurrent medical condition.

Many nonprescription medications are taken PRN. Document the potential use (e.g., 1 to 2 tablets every 4 to 6 hours PRN for headache) as well as the actual use (e.g., 2 tablets twice a day 1 day a month for headache). Quantification of the exact amount of medication taken by the patient may be difficult but is important; do not accept imprecise descriptive terms. One approach to quantifying the amount of nonprescription medication taken by the patient is to ask the patient how often he or she buys a new supply of the medication (e.g., 1 bottle weekly, monthly, yearly). This information provides an indirect assessment of the amount of medication the patient actually takes.

PAST NONPRESCRIPTION MEDICATIONS

Obtain as much information as possible about past nonprescription medications, including name and description, dosage, prescribed or recommended and actual dosing schedule, dates and duration of therapy, reason for taking, reason for stopping, and outcome. Knowledge of past nonprescription regimens gives the pharmacist insight regarding past medical problems or attempts to treat current medical problems. As with prescription medications, patients are unlikely to remember all of these details for past medications. Document the details the patient can remember; avoid excessive "grilling" of the patient.

ALTERNATIVE REMEDIES

Approximately 7% of Americans take alternative remedies (e.g., herbal remedies, megavitamins, homeopathic medicine, folk remedies),[7] also known as *complementary medicines*. However, the majority of people do not discuss these therapies with their physicians.[7] Many of these remedies interact with traditional medicines; some have significant side effects. Therefore it is important to document the use of these products.

Obtain a complete description of current and past alternative remedies used. Document the name and dosage of the product, dosing schedule, duration of therapy, reason the patient is taking the product, start and stop dates or approximate duration and timing of use, and outcome of therapy. As with many prescription and nonprescription medications, many alternative remedies are taken PRN; quantification of the exact amount of product consumed by the patient may be difficult. However, quantification is important; do not accept imprecise descriptive terms. As with prescription and nonprescription drugs, ask the patient how often he or she buys a new supply of the product to gain an indirect assessment of the amount of product taken by the patient.

MEDICATION ALLERGIES

Many health care professionals fail to differentiate between a drug allergy and an adverse drug reaction. The term *allergy* indicates hypersensitivity to specific substances. Drug-induced allergic reactions include anaphylaxis, contact dermatitis, and serum sickness. Once a medication allergy is documented for a patient, it is highly unlikely that the patient will receive the medication or a similar medication again. If the reaction was a manageable or acceptable adverse reaction rather than an allergic reaction, the patient may be unnecessarily denied access to potentially useful medications.

The identification of true medication allergies may be difficult. A useful first step is to ask patients whether they are allergic to any medications and then probe for the details of the problem depending on the response. Ask patients if they have ever experienced rashes or breathing problems after taking any medications. Patients may not correlate a rash with an allergy, so it is important to probe for these details.

After a medication has been identified as the cause of an allergic reaction, ask the patient to provide details regarding the time or date of the allergic reaction, any interventions instituted to manage the reaction, and whether the patient has received the medication since first experiencing the allergic reaction. Ask whether medications in similar drug classes have been taken without the occurrence of a similar reaction.

Advise patients who have documented life-threatening allergic reactions about programs such as the Medic Alert program, which provides patients with necklaces and bracelets engraved with patient-specific allergy information.

ADVERSE DRUG REACTIONS

Adverse drug reactions are unwanted pharmacologic effects associated with medications. Examples of adverse drug reactions include drowsiness from first-generation antihistamines, constipation from codeine-containing medications, nausea from theophylline, and diarrhea from ampicillin. The patient may identify some adverse drug reactions during the discussion of medication allergies. Ask patients whether they have ever taken a medication they would rather not take again. This question often elicits specific descriptions of adverse reactions the patient has experienced. Determine the name of the medication, the dosage, the reason the patient was taking the medication, the date of the reaction, the details of the adverse reaction, and the way the patient dealt with the reaction (e.g., discontinued the medication, decreased the dosage of the medication, took another medication to treat the adverse reaction).

COMPLIANCE

One of the goals of the medication history interview is to determine whether the patient is compliant with prescribed or recommended medication regimens. Knowledge regarding patient compliance is useful in evaluating the effectiveness of prescribed or recommended medication regimens. Medications may be ineffective if the patient does not comply with the prescribed or recommended regimen. Noncompliance may result in additional diagnostic evaluations, procedures, hospitalizations, and unnecessary combination medication regimens.

Compliance is difficult to determine through direct questioning. Patients know they should be compliant. When confronted by an authority figure, patients most likely will say they are compliant even if they are not. Therefore evaluate the patient's compliance by gentle probing throughout the interview. Clues about compliance may be obtained through patients' descriptions of how they take their prescribed medications. Many patients can describe their medication routines in detail (e.g., setting out a day's worth of doses in the morning, lining up the bottles in a special location, crossing off dates on a calendar); other patients may not be able to describe any sort of routine or even recall the color or shape of the medication. Patients who can convincingly describe their medication routines are more likely to be compliant than patients who can provide only vague and general descriptions of their medications and routines.

Sympathetic confrontation may help the pharmacist obtain information regarding patient compliance. If the pharmacist acknowledges that the dosage regimen is complex and difficult to follow or that taking medication regularly is hard, patients are more likely to be truthful when describing their difficulties with complying with the regimens. Remain nonjudgmental when assessing patient compliance; this attitude encourages the patient to trust the pharmacist and tell the truth about adherence to prescribed medication regimens.

THE DIFFICULT INTERVIEW

Obtaining medication history information from patients is sometimes difficult. Some patients are especially difficult to interview. Recalcitrant patients, verbose patients, confused patients, patients whose command of the English language is limited, patients with hearing impairments, patients with aphasia, impatient patients, and patients hospitalized in isolation rooms all may be difficult to interview. Although these types of patients may intimidate even the most experienced interviewer, it is important to obtain accurate medication histories from them.

Many interventions are possible. The best approach for recalcitrant or verbose patients is to exert firm control of the interview and ask directed questions to draw information from the recalcitrant patient and redirect the verbose patient. The confused or aphasic patient may be unable to provide any specific information. In this situation, interview family members and friends of the patient. Interpreters are available for many foreign languages in most institutions; take advantage of these resources. Enhance communication with patients with hearing impairments by ensuring that the patient's hearing aid (if any) is turned on, by speaking clearly and distinctly, and by sharing written information with the patient. Remind the impatient patient of the usefulness of an accurate medication history and try to obtain the history efficiently and in a reasonable amount of time.

The process for interviewing patients in isolation rooms (e.g., respiratory isolation, enteric isolation, infectious disease isolation) is the same as is the process for interviewing any other hospitalized patient with the exception that precautions (e.g., masks, gowns, gloves) must be taken; these precautions usually are posted outside the patient's room. Be aware that these precautions may present barriers to communication. Most isolation patients are especially eager to be interviewed because isolation prevents much of the casual human contact that routinely takes place with institutionalized patients.

QUESTIONING TECHNIQUES

Ask open-ended questions at the start of the interview and then move to more direct and targeted questions as the interview proceeds. For example, a good opening question is to ask the patient to describe any medications taken daily. This question allows the patient to discuss his or her medication routines and provides the pharmacist with clues regarding lines of targeted questioning to be pursued later in the interview. An example of a more direct and targeted question is to ask the patient to describe the size, shape, and color of the medication regularly taken. Every patient is different, so be flexible and guide the patient through the interview.

Avoid asking leading questions, multiple questions, and excessive yes/no questions. Leading questions—such as "Does your tuberculosis medication turn your urine red?"—may make the patient think the medication is supposed to turn the urine red and that something is wrong with them if their urine is not red. Probe for these types of medication-related effects by asking more general questions—such as "How are you tolerating your tuberculosis medications? Have you noticed anything different or unusual since you started taking the medication?" Avoid the trap of getting into a pattern of asking a series of rapid-fire questions without giving the patient time to answer. Give the patient ample time to address each question before asking another question. Getting into a pattern of asking a series of yes/no questions also is very easy, especially toward the end of the interview, when the pharmacist asks specific and targeted questions. Such a series might include questions such as, "Do you take anything for headache? Do you take anything for your eyes? Do you take anything for your heart? Do you take anything for your breathing? Do you take anything when you have a cold? Have you ever taken penicillin?" These types of rapid-fire yes/no questions create one-sided conversations and may diminish the flow of information from the patient. Encourage patients to talk about their experiences with medications.

DOCUMENTING THE MEDICATION HISTORY

The details of the medication history are documented in writing and communicated to the health care team. Many standardized patient profile forms have specific areas for the documentation of this information. Some institutions use standardized

Medication History

Patient: John Smith		**Date:** 1/31/03

Pharmacist: Jane Doe, Pharm.D., RPh

Date of Admission: 01/31/03	**Room:** 1221B	**ID Number:** 8963011
DOB: 12/03/41	**Gender:** M	**Height:** 5'11"	**Weight:** 185 lbs.

Current Prescription Medications (nonproprietary/proprietary names, start date, dose, schedule, indication):
Disopyramide (Norpace) 200 mg po q 6 h × 2 wks "for heart", is not working
Captopril (Capoten) 25 mg po TID × about 10 years for HTN; control BP
Warfarin (Coumadin) 5 mg po qd; started 12/15/02; to "prevent clots"
Digoxin (Lanoxin) 0.25 mg po qd; started 12/15/93; to "slow down heart"

Past Prescription Medications (nonproprietary/proprietary names, start/stop dates, dose, schedule, indication):
Quinidine gluconate (Quinaglute) 324-648 mg po TID in 12/02 for "rapid heart"; exact dates unclear; did not work
Procainamide (Procan) 500 mg po q 6 h × 3 days in 12/02 for "rapid heart"; exact dates unclear; did not work

Current Nonprescription Medications (proprietary/nonproprietary names, start date, dose, schedule, indication):
Simethicone (Mylicon) unknown dose (described as one small white tablet) PRN gas; rare use; buys one box every couple of years; has used for "years"; very effective
Acetaminophen (Tylenol) 650 mg PRN HA; rare use; takes 1-2 doses about 6 times a year for "many years"; very effective

Past Nonprescription Medications (proprietary/nonproprietary names, start/stop dates, dose, schedule, indication):
EC ASA (Ecotrin) 325 mg po daily for 5 years to "prevent heart attacks"; stopped 12/15/02 when warfarin (Coumadin) started

Alternative Remedies (proprietary/nonproprietary names, start/stop dates, dose, schedule, indication):
Echinacea 2 capsules BID with food for several days when he has a cold for the last three years; takes for the duration of the cold (1-2 weeks); has 2-3 colds/year; effective

Allergies (proprietary/nonproprietary names, dates, description of event, treatment):
NKDA

Adverse Drug Reactions:
None

Social History (tobacco, alcohol, illicit drugs, marital status, occupation, housing):
Accountant; lives in own home with wife
+ Tobacco (1 ppd × 40 yrs; 40 pk-yrs)
+ Alcohol (one six-pack of beer per week × 40 yrs)
Denies use of illicit drugs

Dietary Information (restrictions, supplements, stimulants):
Restrictions: NAS diet × "years"
Supplements: None
Stimulants: None

Assessment of Patient Compliance:
Patient knows his medications and seems to be compliant. He is eager to have his atrial fibrillation under control and is willing to try any medication.

Plan:
Continue the digoxin (Lanoxin), warfarin (Coumadin), and captopril (Capoten). Check the most recent INR and serum digoxin (Lanoxin) concentration; adjust as necessary. Proceed with propafenone (Rythmol) as planned. Monitor for increased serum digoxin (Lanoxin) concentrations when propafenone (Rythmol) is added and adjust the dioxin dose as necessary. Consider alternative medications such as low-dose amiodarone (Amrinone) if propafenone (Rythmol) or electrical cardioversion does not convert to NSR. Advise the patient about the risks associated with echinacea.

Figure 3-1
Medication History—Standardized Form.
Standardized forms are easy to fill out but are inflexible.

medication history forms that are filled out, signed, and placed in the patient medical record (Figure 3-1). These standardized forms are relatively easy to complete and are easy to scan for specific information. However, standardized forms are inflexible and may not contain adequate space for documentation of patient-specific information. Document the medication history in the patient record using either the SOAP format (Subjective, Objective, Assessment, Plan) (Figure 3-2) or freestyle format (Figure 3-3) if standardized forms are not available. The SOAP format organizes the medication history information into four sections: subjective data, objective data, assessment, and plan; the information is well organized, but it is hard for readers to scan the document for specific information. The freestyle format organizes the infor-

---

01/31/03   **Medication History**

S: "Rapid heart"

O: John Smith is a 62 y/o WM (DOB 12/03/41) with HTN × 10 yrs and recent-onset atrial fibrillation noted on routine physical exam last month. He failed trials of quinidine (Quinaglute), disopyramide (Norpace), and procainamide (Procan). He is admitted for a trial of propafenone (Rythmol). Electrical cardioversion is planned if propafenone (Rythmol) does not work. He is 5'11" and weighs 185 lbs. He has NKDA and no known adverse drug reactions. He smokes 1 ppd × 40 yrs (40 pk-yr hx). He drinks a six-pack of beer per week and has done so for 40 yrs. He denies illicit drug use. He is an accountant and lives in his own home with his wife. He limits his salt intake (no added salt at the table); no dietary supplements or stimulants.

His current prescription medications include disopyramide (Norpace) 200 mg po every 6 hours × 2 weeks "for heart", captopril (Capoten) 25 mg po TID for about 10 years for HTN, warfarin (Coumadin) 5 mg daily to "prevent clots" (started 12/15/02) and digoxin (Lanoxin) 0.25 mg po daily to "slow down heart" (started 12/15/02). The disopyramide (Norpace) is not working. The captopril (Capoten) is controlling his BP. His past prescription medications include quinidine gluconate (Quinaglute) 324-648 mg po TID in 12/02 for "rapid heart"; exact dates and doses unclear; did not work, procainamide (Procan) 500 mg po every 6 hours × 3 days in 12/02 for "rapid heart"; taken after quinidine gluconate (Quinaglute); exact dates unclear; did not work.

His current nonprescription medications include simethicone (Mylicon) unknown dose (one small white tablet) PRN gas (buys one box every couple of years; very effective), acetaminophen (Tylenol) 650 mg PRN HA (takes 1-2 doses about 6 times per year and has done so for "many years"; very effective). Used to take EC ASA (Ecotrin) 325 mg po daily for about 5 years to prevent heart attacks until it was stopped 12/15/02 when warfarin (Coumadin) was started. He has not taken any other nonprescription medications.

JS takes echinacea 2 capsules BID with food for several days when he has a cold; takes for the duration of the cold (1-2 weeks); has 2-3 colds/year. He has taken echinacea for the last 3 years and says it is very effective.

A: JS has an excellent knowledge regarding the medication he has taken. He is eager to have his atrial fibrillation under control and claims to take all medication exactly as prescribed. His blood pressure is adequately controlled with the current regimen.

P: Continue the digoxin (Lanoxin), warfarin (Coumadin), and captopril (Capoten). Check the most recent INR and serum digoxin (Lanoxin) concentration; adjust as necessary. Proceed with propafenone (Rythmol) as planned. Monitor for increased serum digoxin (Lanoxin) concentration when propafenone (Rythmol) is added and adjust the digoxin (Lanoxin) as necessary. If propafenone (Rythmol) or electrical cardioversion are ineffective, consider a trial of alternative medications such as low-dose amiodarone (Amrinone). Counsel about the risks associated with echinacea.

                                                 Jane Doe, Pharm.D., RPh

Figure 3-2
Medication History—SOAP Format.
The SOAP format produces well-organized information, but it may be difficult for others to locate specific information.

mation into whatever structure the pharmacist thinks best for the information. It is easy to write a medication history in a freestyle format, but finding specific details may be difficult; important information is more likely to be left out in this format than with other formats.

01/31/03   **Medication History**

John Smith is a 62 y/o WM (DOB 12/03/41) with a PMH significant for HTN × 10 years and recent-onset atrial fibrillation described as "rapid heart" noted on routine physical exam in 12/02. He was initially started on a trial of quinidine (Quinaglute), which failed to convert him back to NSR. Disopyramide (Norpace) and procainamide (Procan) were tried but also failed to convert him to NSR. He is being admitted for a trial of propafenone (Rythmol); electrical cardioversion will be tried if propafenone fails. 5'11", 185 lbs.

SH: Accountant; lives in own home with wife; + tobacco (1 ppd × 40 yrs; 40 pk-yrs); + alcohol (one six-pack of beer per week × 40 yrs); denies illicit drugs

Dietary: NAS; no stimulants; no supplements

Allergies: NKDA

ADRs: None

Current Prescription Medications:
> Disopyramide (Norpace) 200 mg po q 6 h × 2 wks "for heart", is not working
> Captopril (Capoten) 25 mg po TID × about 10 years for HTN; control BP
> Warfarin (Coumadin) 5 mg po qd; started 12/15/02; to "prevent clots"
> Digoxin (Lanoxin) 0.25 mg po qd; started 12/15/93; to "slow down heart"

Past Prescription Medications:
> Quinidine gluconate (Quinaglute) 324-648 mg po TID in 12/02 for "rapid heart"; exact dates unclear; did not work
> Procainamide (Procan) 500 mg po q 6 h × 3 days in 12/02 for "rapid heart"; exact dates unclear; did not work

Current Nonprescription Medications:
> Simethicone (Mylicon) unknown dose (described as one small white tablet) PRN gas; rare use; buys one box every couple of years; has used for "years"; very effective
> Acetaminophen (Tylenol) 650 mg PRN HA; rare use; takes 1-2 doses about 6 times a year for "many years"; very effective

Past Nonprescription Medications:
> EC ASA (Ecotrin) 325 mg po daily for 5 years to "prevent heart attacks"; stopped 12/15/02 when warfarin (Coumadin) started

Alternative Remedies:
> Echinacea 2 capsules BID with food for several days when he has a cold for 3 years; takes for the duration of the cold (1-2 weeks); has 2-3 colds/year; effective

JS knows his medications well and appears to be very compliant. He is eager to have his atrial fibrillation under control and is willing to try any medication. Continue captopril (Capoten), digoxin (Lanoxin), and coumadin (Warfarin) but check the most recent INR and serum digoxin concentration and adjust the dosages as necessary. Proceed with propafenone (Rythmol) as planned. Monitor for increased serum digoxin concentrations with the addition of propafenone (Rythmol). If propafenone (Rythmol) or electrical conversion do not control his atrial fibrillation, consider a trial of alternate medications such as low-dose amiodarone (Amrinone).

                                                        Jane Doe, Pharm.D., RPh

---

Figure 3-3
Medication History—Freestyle Format.
The freestyle format makes writing specific information easy but finding information difficult.

Regardless of the format used to document the information, it is important to document every component of the medication history. Documenting that the patient is not taking any current prescription drugs is as important as documenting that the patient is taking a long list of current prescription drugs. Document all the details. Write clearly. Document both the *nonproprietary* drug name (the name intended for unrestricted public use; sometimes referred to as the generic drug name) and the *proprietary* drug name (the legally trademarked name) when the patient refers to a medication by the proprietary name. Document just the nonproprietary drug name if the patient refers to the drug by the nonproprietary name. For example, if the patient says she takes Avandia, document the proprietary name "Avandia" and the nonproprietary name "rosiglitazone." If the patient says he takes "pseudoephedrine," document the nonproprietary name "pseudoephedrine." Checklists may be useful (Box 3-5).

BOX 3-5

Medication History Checklist

EACH OF THE FOLLOWING DETAILS IS INCLUDED:
- ❏ The history is written in black ink.
- ❏ The date and time of the interview are noted.
- ❏ The history includes an appropriate heading (e.g., Medication History).
- ❏ The history is signed (and cosigned if written by a student).
- ❏ All medications are referred to by nonproprietary and (if applicable) proprietary names; a complete description of the dosage form is provided if name not known.
- ❏ The start date is noted for all medications.
- ❏ The stop date is noted for all past medications.
- ❏ The dosage and interval are noted for all medications.
- ❏ The indication for each medication is noted.
- ❏ The actual use of each PRN medication is noted ("as needed" and "occasional" are not acceptable descriptions).
- ❏ The actual use of each social and recreational drug is noted ("as needed" and "occasional" are not acceptable descriptions).
- ❏ The details of all adverse reactions are noted (drug, date, reaction, treatment).
- ❏ The details of all medication allergies are noted (drug, date, reaction, treatment).

EACH OF THE FOLLOWING COMPONENTS IS INCLUDED:
- ❏ Patient demographics
- ❏ Current prescription medications
- ❏ Current nonprescription medications
- ❏ Current alternative remedies
- ❏ Past prescription medications
- ❏ Past nonprescription medications
- ❏ Past alternative remedies
- ❏ Medication allergies
- ❏ Adverse drug reactions
- ❏ Dietary information
- ❏ Social drug information
- ❏ Assessment of compliance

SELF-ASSESSMENT QUESTIONS

1. Which of the following is a disadvantage of reviewing all available information about a patient before interviewing the patient?
   a. The pharmacist feels more comfortable.
   b. The pharmacist is prepared to address specific issues.
   c. The pharmacist may be too focused and overlook important issues.
   d. The pharmacist is completely unbiased about all aspects of the history.
   e. The pharmacist feels more intimidated.

2. During a patient interview the pharmacist observes that the patient's clothing has a predominance of Velcro-type fastenings. This may indicate which of the following?
   a. Photosensitivity
   b. Recent weight loss
   c. Recent weight gain
   d. Loss of manual dexterity
   e. Hypertension

3. Demographic patient information includes all of the following *except*:
   a. Age
   b. Height
   c. Weight
   d. Ethnic origin
   e. Dietary restrictions

4. A patient states that he has smoked 2 packs of cigarettes a day for 30 years. What is the patient's pack-year smoking history?
   a. 2 pack-years
   b. 15 pack-years
   c. 30 pack-years
   d. 60 pack-years
   e. 90 pack-years

5. Current prescription information includes all of the following *except*:
   a. The name and description of the drug
   b. The date or time the medication was stopped
   c. The dosage of the drug
   d. The prescribed and actual dosing schedule
   e. The date or time the medication was started

6. What information is documented regarding a suspected medication allergy?
   a. The date or time the reaction occurred
   b. The interventions performed to manage the reaction
   c. Whether the patient has received similar medications
   d. All of the above
   e. None of the above

7. Which of the following questioning techniques is *least* likely to result in an accurate assessment of patient compliance?
   a. Directly questioning the patient
   b. Gently probing
   c. Confronting the patient sympathetically
   d. Being nonjudgmental during questioning
   e. Asking the patient to describe the daily routine

8. In general, which of the following types of questions should be avoided when interviewing patients?
   a. Leading questions
   b. Multiple questions
   c. Excessive yes/no questions
   d. All of the above
   e. None of the above

9. Which of the following is the best approach to interviewing verbose patients?
   a. Asking directed questions
   b. Interviewing family members
   c. Using an interpreter
   d. Speaking slowly and loudly
   e. Interviewing friends

10. Which one of the following is a disadvantage of documenting a medication history using the freestyle format?
   a. The format is inflexible.
   b. Scanning the document for specific details is difficult.
   c. Space may not be available for all patient information.
   d. All of the above
   e. None of the above

References

1. Wilson RS, Kabat HF: Pharmacist initiated patient drug histories, Am J Hosp Pharm 28:49-53, 1971.
2. Covington TR, Pfeiffer FG: The pharmacist-acquired medication history, Am J Hosp Pharm 29:692-695, 1972.
3. Zakus GE et al: Teaching interviewing for pediatrics, J Med Ed 51:325-331, 1976.
4. Lipkin M Jr, Quill TE, Napodano RJ: The medical interview: a core curriculum for residencies in internal medicine, Ann Intern Med 100:277-284, 1984.
5. Preven DW et al: Interviewing skills of first-year medical students, J Med Ed 61:842-844, 1986.
6. Fitzgerald FT, Tierney LM Jr: The bedside Sherlock Holmes, West J Med 137:169-175, 1982.
7. Eisenberg DM et al: Unconventional medicine in the United States. Prevalence, costs, and patterns of use, N Engl J Med 328:246-252, 1993.

Physical Assessment Skills

CHAPTER 4

Learning Objectives

- List the four fundamental physical assessment techniques and describe how to perform each of the techniques.
- Identify the components of the stethoscope, ophthalmoscope, and otoscope and state how each instrument is used to assess patients.
- Describe how to use a tuning fork and a reflex hammer.
- Describe how to assess each of the major organ systems.
- Define common physical assessment terms.
- Interpret common physical assessment abbreviations.

*L*aboratory data, data obtained during a patient medication history interview, and information obtained from the physical examination are used to assess patient response to drug and nondrug therapy. Although the need for hands-on proficiency in specific physical assessment skills varies according to the type of patient care setting, all pharmacists need a basic understanding of these skills. At a minimum, all pharmacists must know common physical assessment abbreviations (Table 4-1) and understand the meaning of specific physical assessment findings documented by other health care professionals. Pharmacists in some clinical settings (e.g., ambulatory care clinics) routinely assess patients using a variety of physical assessment skills. Although the practice settings requiring proficiency in a broad range of physical assessment skills are currently relatively few in number, the need for these skills continues to grow as pharmacists assume more direct patient care responsibilities.

This chapter introduces the pharmacist to the processes, techniques, and components of the physical examination. However, physical examination is a complex process that requires significant effort and experience to master. Pharmacists interested in learning more about the physical examination should refer to one or more of the excellent in-depth physical examination textbooks available in medical libraries and bookstores. In addition, an increasing number of hands-on continuing education physical assessment courses are available for pharmacists.

TABLE 4-1

Common Physical Assessment Abbreviations

Abbreviation	Meaning
Abdominal	
Abd	Abdomen
BRBPR	Bright red blood per rectum
BS	Bowel sounds
CM	Costal margin
HJR	Hepatojugular reflux
HSM	Hepatosplenomegaly
LCM	Left costal margin
LLQ	Left lower quadrant
LUQ	Left upper quadrant
NABS	Normal active bowel sounds
NTND	Nontender, nondistended
RCM	Right costal margin
RLQ	Right lower quadrant
RUQ	Right upper quadrant
Cardiovascular	
AI	Aortic insufficiency
AR	Aortic regurgitation
AS	Aortic stenosis
5ICSMCL	Fifth intercostal space midclavicular line
CV	Cardiovascular
JVD	Jugular venous distention
JVP	Jugular venous pressure
LLSB	Left lower sternal border
m	Murmur
MAP	Mean arterial pressure
MR	Mitral regurgitation
mrg	Murmurs, rubs, gallops
MS	Mitral stenosis
MVP	Mitral valve prolapse
NSR	Normal sinus rhythm
OS	Opening snap
PMI	Point of maximal impulse
RRR	Regular rate and rhythm
S_1	First heart sound
S_2	Second heart sound
S_3	Third heart sound
S_4	Fourth heart sound
SEM	Systolic ejection murmur
USB	Upper sternal border

Continued

TABLE 4-1

Common Physical Assessment Abbreviations—cont'd

Abbreviation	Meaning
Extremities	
AKA	Above-knee amputation
BKA	Below-knee amputation
CCE	Cyanosis, clubbing, and edema
CVA	Costovertebral angle
CVAT	Costovertebral angle tenderness
DP	Dorsalis pedis
FROM	Full range of motion
LE	Lower extremity
LLE	Left lower extremity
LUE	Left upper extremity
PT	Popliteal
RLE	Right lower extremity
ROM	Range of motion
RUE	Right upper extremity
Tr	Trace
UE	Upper extremity
General	
ABW	Actual body weight
AF	Asian female
AM	Asian male
A&O × 3	Awake and oriented to person, place, and time
A&P	Auscultation and percussion
A&W	Alive and well
BF	Black female
BM	Black male
BP	Blood pressure
BPM	Beats per minute; breaths per minute
Bx	Biopsy
DBP	Diastolic blood pressure
HF	Hispanic female
HM	Hispanic male
HR	Heart rate
IBW	Ideal body weight
LBW	Lean body weight
AAF	African-American female
AAM	African-American male
NAD	No acute distress; no apparent disease
PE	Physical examination
PPD	Packs per day
SBP	Systolic blood pressure

TABLE 4-1

Common Physical Assessment Abbreviations—cont'd

Abbreviation	Meaning
T	Temperature
$T_{(a)}$	Temperature, axillary
$T_{(po)}$	Temperature, oral
$T_{(R)}$	Temperature, rectal
$T_{(T)}$	Temperature, tympanic
VS	Vital signs
VSS	Vital signs stable
WDWN	Well developed, well nourished
WF	White female
WM	White male
WNL	Within normal limits
Y/O	Years old
Head, Eyes, Ears, Nose, and Throat	
C/D	Cup-to-disc ratio
EOMI	Extraocular muscles intact
HEENT	Head, eyes, ears, nose, and throat
IOP	Intraocular pressure
NCAT	Normocephalic, atraumatic
NR	Nonreactive
OD	Right eye
OS	Left eye
PERRLA	Pupils equal, round, and reactive to light and accommodation
SCM	Sternocleidomastoid
SHEENT	Skin, head, eyes, ears, nose, and throat
TM	Tympanic membrane
Neurologic	
AC	Air conduction
AC > BC	Air conduction greater than bone conduction
Bab	Babinski reflex
BC	Bone conduction
BC > AC	Bone conduction greater than air conduction
CN	Cranial nerve
CN II-XII	Cranial nerves II through XII (2 through 12)
DTR	Deep tendon reflex
FTN	Finger-to-nose
HTS	Heel-to-shin
MMSE	Mini-Mental Status Examination
MS	Mental status
MSE	Mental status examination
NM	Neuromuscular
PP	Pinprick
RAM	Rapid alternating movements

Continued

TABLE 4-1

Common Physical Assessment Abbreviations—cont'd

Abbreviation	Meaning
Pulmonary	
AP	Anteroposterior
BS	Breath sounds
CTA	Clear to auscultation
E→A	Egophony
LLL	Left lower lobe
LUL	Left upper lobe
PA	Posteroanterior
RLL	Right lower lobe
RML	Right middle lobe
RR	Respiratory rate
RUL	Right upper lobe

THE PROCESS

The examination, usually conducted from the patient's right side, follows a generally accepted sequence that minimizes the number of changes in position by the patient and clinician (Box 4-1). It is important to respect the patient's privacy and minimize patient discomfort and embarrassment throughout the examination. The scope of the examination varies depending on the patient's illness and its severity. For example, a thorough and detailed examination of all organ systems is required for a severely ill patient with multiple complaints; subsequent examinations may target specific organ system, with perfunctory assessment (if any) of other organ systems. The usual neurologic examination is a simple screening examination unless otherwise indicated.

INSPECTION, PALPATION, PERCUSSION, AND AUSCULTATION TECHNIQUES

The physical examination consists of a detailed patient evaluation using the four fundamental techniques of inspection, percussion, palpation, and auscultation (IPPA). *Inspection* denotes visual surveillance. For example, inspect the skin for color and the presence of lesions, visible trauma, or other abnormalities. *Percussion* determines the density of a specific area or part of the body. Create a percussion note either by tapping the body directly with the distal end of a finger (direct percussion) or by tapping a finger placed on the body (indirect percussion) (Figure 4-1); only the finger being struck touches the body. The resultant sound is described using one of four percussion notes: resonant, dull, tympanic, or flat. These percussion notes are distinguishable with percussion over areas of the body that normally produce the notes (i.e., percussion over normal lung tissue produces a resonant, hollow note; percussion over solid organs such as the liver produces a dull note; percussion over the stomach produces a tympanic note; and percussion over large muscles such as the thigh produces flat notes). *Palpation* consists of using the hands to feel areas

BOX 4-1

The Usual Physical Assessment Sequence

1. Vital signs	7. Nose	14. Extremities
2. Appearance and behavior	8. Mouth	15. Back and spine
	9. Neck	16. Nervous system
3. Skin	10. Breasts	17. Mental status
4. Head	11. Chest and lungs	18. Genitalia and rectum
5. Eyes	12. Heart	
6. Ears	13. Abdomen	

that cannot be seen; palpation can be performed with the fingertips, palm, or back of the hand. Use the back of the hand to assess temperature and the fingertips to feel the lower edge of the liver and the spleen tip. *Auscultation* consists of listening either directly with the ear or indirectly with the aid of a device (typically a stethoscope) to sounds that arise spontaneously from the body (e.g., breath sounds, heart sounds, bowel sounds, bruits).

EQUIPMENT

Several pieces of equipment are required for the physical examination (Table 4-2). The stethoscope, an important auscultatory tool, consists of two ear pieces angled at the same angle as the ear canal, rubber tubing, and a head with either a diaphragm or a

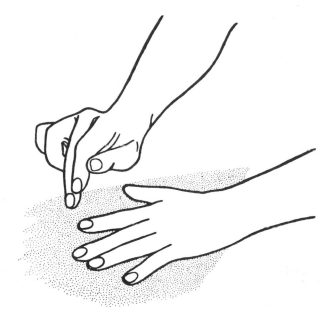

Figure 4-1
Percussion.
Technique for indirect percussion. Only the pleximeter finger contacts the body. (From Wilkins RL, Sheldon RL, Krider SJ, editors: *Clinical assessment in respiratory care*, ed 4, St Louis, 2000, Mosby.)

TABLE 4-2

Physical Assessment Equipment

Equipment	Purpose
Flashlight	Assess pupillary reflexes; aid in the inspection of the oropharynx and skin
Ophthalmoscope	Perform funduscopic examination
Otoscope	Assess external ear canal and tympanic membrane
Tongue depressor	Inspect oropharynx
Watch (digital or sweep second hand)	Assess heart and respiratory rate
Thermometer	Obtain body temperature
Stethoscope	Assess cardiovascular, pulmonary, and abdominal systems
Sphygmomanometer	Obtain blood pressure
Reflex hammer	Assess neurologic function
Tuning fork	Assess neurologic function

bell and a diaphragm (a dual-headed stethoscope) (Figure 4-2). The bell transmits low-frequency sounds; the diaphragm accentuates high-frequency sounds. Stethoscopes are available in a variety of styles and prices, including electronically amplified stethoscopes. Although the choice of style (e.g., Sprague Rappaport type with dual tubing, Littman type with a single tube) depends on personal preference, quality is important. Higher-quality stethoscopes transmit sounds more efficiently and are more durable than cheaper models. The earpieces should fit the ear canals snugly and comfortably; the goal is for the sound to be transmitted from the patient to the eardrum through an unbroken system. Most quality stethoscopes come with several different sizes and shapes of ear tips, enabling the user to select the best fitting and most comfortable tips.

The ophthalmoscope consists of a head and a handle (Figure 4-3). The head contains viewing lenses and beam selection controls. The viewing lens control (lens wheel) is used to focus the instrument. Positive diopters (black or green numbers depending on the manufacturer) are used for nearsighted eyes; negative diopters (red numbers) are used for farsighted eyes. The beam control wheel is used to select the aperture (beam); aperture selection depends on the structure being assessed (Table 4-3). The light intensity is adjustable on some ophthalmoscopes.

The otoscope consists of a head and a handle (Figure 4-4). The head consists of a speculum and magnifying glass and can be rotated up and down in several positions. Disposable speculum covers are available in a variety of sizes to fit most ear canals. Most otoscopes and ophthalmoscopes are available as interchangeable heads that fit the same handle.

SKIN

The skin is evaluated using inspection and palpation.

Inspection.   Inspect the skin for color (pallor, cyanosis, redness, yellowness), lesions, trauma, or other abnormalities. Inspect the nails and nail beds for clubbing, cyanosis, or trauma. Note the distribution, amount, and texture of the body hair.

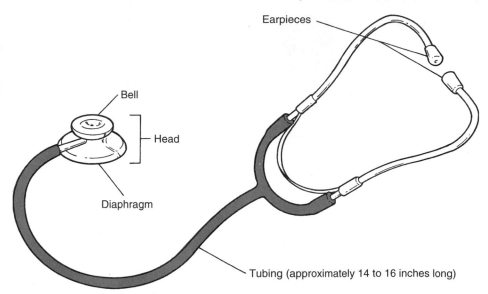

Figure 4-2
The Stethoscope.
Components of the stethoscope.

Palpation.   Palpate the skin for turgor (hydration status), moistness, temperature (warm, cool), texture (rough, smooth), thickness (thick, thin), mobility (immobile, mobile, hypermobile), and edema. Assess skin turgor by pulling up and quickly releasing a fold of skin. In a well-hydrated patient, the skin quickly returns to normal; it takes longer for the skin to return to normal if the patient is dehydrated (tenting). Describe lesions according to location, type, color, shape, size, grouping, and pattern. Assess edema by pressing the tips of one or two fingers into the skin and noting how long the indentation remains after the fingers are removed. A plus scale (1+, 2+, 3+, 4+) is used to quantify the edema, with 4+ denoting the most long-lasting indentations.

TERMINOLOGY
Lesions
  Primary Lesions
    bulla: A large (>1 cm), circumscribed, elevated lesion containing serous fluid, such as blistering from second-degree burns
    ecchymosis: A large (>1 cm) hemorrhage, commonly known as a *bruise*
    macule: A small (<1 cm), circumscribed, flat, discolored lesion, such as a freckle or flat nevus
    nodule: A large (>1 cm), solid lesion that may be below, even with, or above the surface of the skin
    papule: A small (<1 cm), elevated, solid lesion, such as a wart
    patch: An area containing discolored, circumscribed, and flat or elevated groups of lesions, such as a measles rash

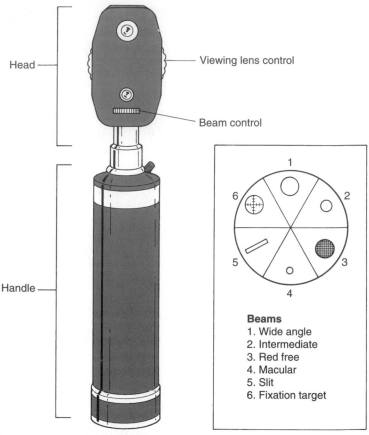

Figure 4-3
The Ophthalmoscope.
Components of the ophthalmoscope.

TABLE 4-3

Ophthalmoscope Apertures

Aperture	Use
Wide angle	Assess dilated pupils
Intermediate	Assess undilated pupils and details of small areas
Red free	Assess retinal vessels
Macular	Assess macula
Slit	Assess cornea, anterior chamber, and elevations or depressions in the fundus
Fixation target	Assess eccentric fixation

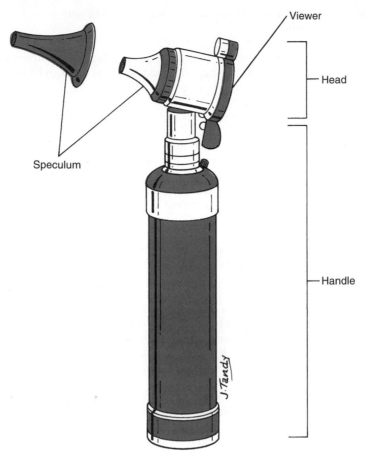

Viewer

Head

Speculum

Handle

Figure 4-4
The Otoscope.
Components of the otoscope.

petechia: A small (<2 mm) hemorrhage
plaque: A large (>1 cm), circumscribed, elevated, and solid lesion, such as pityriasis rosea
pustule: A circumscribed, elevated lesion of varying size containing pus, such as impetigo
vesicle: A small (<1 cm), circumscribed, elevated lesion containing serous fluid, such as herpes zoster
wheal: An edematous and transitory papule, such as hives
Secondary Lesions
crust: A mass of dried exudate, such as impetigo
excoriation: A scratch mark usually covered with blood or serous crusts
fissure: A linear break in the skin
keloid: A hypertrophic scar

lichenification: Thickening and roughening of the skin with increased visibility of normal skin lines

scale: Dead epidermal cells, such as dandruff

scar: Area in which normal skin tissue has been replaced by connective tissue

ulcer: An irregularly sized and shaped excavation that extends below the dermal skin layer, such as a pressure sore

Other Lesions

comedo (blackhead):   A pilosebaceous follicular plug of sebaceous and keratinous material

milium (whitehead):   A small (1 to 2 mm) nodule with no visible opening

nevus (mole):   A flat or elevated pigmented lesion

Osler's node: A small, raised, discolored, tender lesion on the pads of the fingers and toes associated with bacterial endocarditis

telangiectasias: Dilated superficial blood vessels

Fingernail and Toenail Terms

Beau's lines: Transverse horizontal depressions associated with severe illness

clubbing: Increased angle (>180 degrees) between the base of the nail and the nail bed; associated with chronic arterial desaturation (e.g., chronic obstructive pulmonary disease [COPD])

koilonychia: Spooning of the nails associated with iron deficiency anemia

onycholysis: Separation of the nail from the nail bed associated with trauma, malnutrition, and thyroid disease

splinter hemorrhages: Red or brown linear streaks in the distal extremity of the nail bed; nonspecific

HEAD AND NECK

The structures of the head and neck (skull, scalp, face, neck, nose, ears, mouth and pharynx, and eyes) are evaluated through inspection and palpation; percussion and auscultation are rarely indicated. Visual acuity, hearing, and facial and ophthalmic reflexes are tested when clinically indicated.

SKULL
Inspection.   Inspect the skull for size, contour, shape, and evidence of trauma.

Palpation.   Palpate the skull for lumps, bumps, and evidence of trauma.

HAIR
Inspection.   Inspect the hair for quantity, texture, and distribution.

Palpation.   Palpate the hair for texture (coarse, fine, dry, oily).

SCALP
Inspection.   Inspect the scalp for lesions and scales.

FACE
Inspection.   Inspect the face for expression, symmetry, movement, lesions, and edema.

NECK

Inspection.   Inspect the neck for symmetry, masses, and enlargement of the parotid and submaxillary glands and lymph nodes. Note the position and size of the sternomastoid muscles and the carotid arteries and the position of the trachea.

Palpation.   Palpate the thyroid gland for size, shape, symmetry, tenderness, and nodules. Palpate the lymph nodes (Figure 4-5) for size, shape, mobility, and tenderness.

Auscultation.   Auscultate the thyroid gland if enlarged; a thyroid bruit may be present.

NOSE

Inspection.   Inspect the external nose and nasal cavity for symmetry, inflammation, and lesions. Transilluminate the maxillary sinuses by shining a bright light in the mouth. Normal maxillary sinuses appear as dull-red crescent-shaped glowing areas under each eye. Transilluminate the frontal sinuses by placing a light source under the medial aspect of each eyebrow. Normal frontal sinuses appear as glowing red areas above each eye.

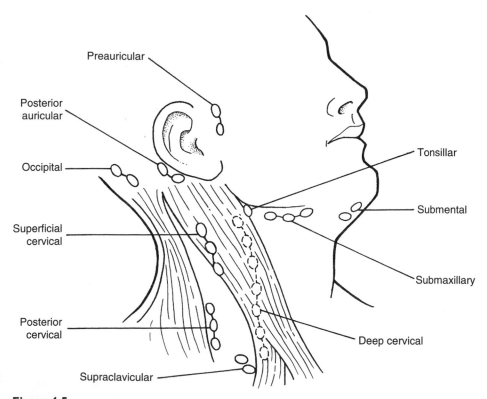

Figure 4-5
Head and Neck Lymph Nodes.
Lymph nodes are located in many regions of the head and neck. (From Delp MH, Manning RT: *Major's physical diagnosis*, ed 9, Philadelphia, 1991, WB Saunders.)

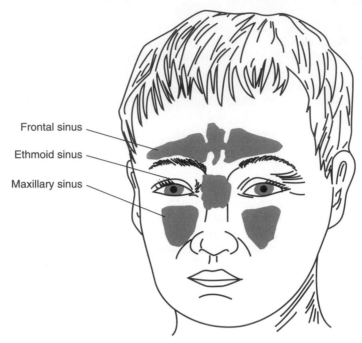

Figure 4-6
The Sinuses.
Frontal, ethmoid, and maxillary sinuses.

Palpation.   Palpate the frontal, ethmoid, and maxillary sinuses for tenderness (Figure 4-6).

EARS
Inspection.   Inspect the external ear for lesions, trauma, size, and contour. Inspect the ear canal and tympanic membranes with the otoscope. Insert the otoscope by tipping the patient's head slightly to the opposite side and gently pulling the auricle up, back, and slightly outward (movement of the auricle and tragus is painful in acute otitis externa). Inspect the canal for foreign bodies (e.g., insects, pieces of toys), discharge, color, and edema. Inspect the tympanic membrane for color, bulging, perforations, and air-fluid levels.

Palpation.   Palpate the external ear for nodules.

HEARING
A general but relatively inaccurate assessment of hearing is obtained by testing, one ear at a time, the ability of the patient to hear a sequence of equally accented syllables (e.g., three-five-two-four) whispered from a distance of a couple of feet. The Rinne test compares bone and air conduction. Place the tip of a vibrating tuning fork (128 or 512 Hz) on the mastoid process behind the ear; this tests bone conduction. Instruct the patient to signal when he or she no longer hears the vibrating tuning fork. Remove the tuning fork from the mastoid process and hold the prongs in front of but not touching the ear canal; this tests air conduction. Normally, air conduction

is better than bone conduction; that is, the patient can hear the vibrating tuning fork when the tuning fork is moved from the mastoid process to in front of the ear canal. To perform the Weber test, place the tip of a vibrating tuning fork on the center of the patient's forehead. Normally, sound is heard equally well in both ears. In conduction loss the sound is heard best in the impaired ear; in unilateral sensorineural hearing loss the sound is heard best in the unimpaired ear.

MOUTH AND PHARYNX

Inspection.   Inspect the lips and mucosa for color, ulcerations, hydration, and lesions. Inspect the teeth and gums for color, bleeding, inflammation, caries, missing teeth, ulcerations, and lesions (Table 4-4). Inspect the hard palate for color, architecture, symmetry, ulcerations, and lesions. Note the movement of the soft palate (elevation and symmetry) when the patient says "ah." Inspect the tonsils and posterior palate for color, edema, ulcerations, exudates, and lesions. Inspect the top, sides, and bottom of the tongue for color, symmetry, ulcerations, and lesions. Note the odor of the breath (e.g., alcohol odor in alcoholic intoxication, urinous odor in uremia, sweetish fruity odor in diabetes mellitus with ketoacidosis, a musty odor [fetor hepaticus] in severe parenchymal liver disease).

EYES

Inspection.   Inspect the external and internal structures of the eyes, and if indicated, assess visual acuity. Obtain a general assessment of visual acuity by asking the patient to read a sentence or two from any printed material (e.g., book, magazine, newspaper). The Snellen eye chart (the chart with the large E on the top line followed by a series of lines with increasingly smaller print) provides a more accurate assessment of visual acuity.

Test the peripheral visual fields with the confrontation technique. Bring a small object (usually your finger) from the patient's visual periphery into the patient's field of vision from several different directions (top, bottom, right side, left side); you can stand in front of or behind the patient.

TABLE 4-4

Oral Lesions

Lesion	Description
Aphthous ulcer (canker sore)	Painful whitish lesion with red border; usually a single lesion
Candidiasis (thrush)	Burning white curdlike lesions with peelable pseudomembranes
Hairy tongue	Painless blackened raised filiform papillae
Herpetic ulcer (cold sore; fever blister)	Painful multiple papules/vesicles; crusting as heals
Leukoplakia	Painless white lesions (look like spilled paint or paint flakes); nonpeelable (precancerous)
Squamous cell carcinoma	Ulcerated single indurated lesion with clean raised borders

Assess the extraocular muscles by having the patient follow the movements of your finger with his or her eyes (keep the head stationary) as the finger is moved in all the six cardinal directions (elevation, depression, adduction, abduction, extorsion, intorsion). The eyes normally follow the finger smoothly and in parallel with the movements; however, far lateral nystagmus may occur normally.

Note the position and alignment of the eyes. If exophthalmos (abnormal protrusion of the eyeball) is observed, inspect the eye from above and note the relationship of the cornea to the eyelids. Inspect the eyelids for color, lesions, edema, and condition of the eyelashes. Inspect the conjunctiva for color and edema and the cornea and lens for opacities. Assess the corneal blink reflex by lightly touching the cornea with a tissue; the normal reflex is to blink.

Inspect the iris and pupil for size, shape, and equality. Assess the iris for abnormal pigments or deposits. Test the pupillary reaction to light by briefly flicking a light on the pupil and noting the direct and consensual (opposite eye) response; both pupils normally constrict in response to the light stimulus. Test the pupillary reaction to accommodation by instructing the patient to focus on an object (usually your finger) from several feet away and then noting the pupillary constriction and convergence ("cross-eyed" response) of the eyes as the object is brought to within a few centimeters in front of the patient's eyes.

Inspect the fundi with the ophthalmoscope. Select the appropriate aperture (see Table 4-3). Hold the ophthalmoscope in the right hand to examine the patient's right eye and in the left hand to examine the patient's left eye; place the index finger on the diopter wheel. Look through the ophthalmoscope with the right eye to examine the patient's right eye; use your left eye to examine the patient's left eye. Prefocus the ophthalmoscope on the wrinkles of your hand placed a few inches in front of your face; this adjusts the ophthalmoscope to your eye and saves time when focusing on the patient's eye. Place the hand not holding the ophthalmoscope on the patient's forehead; this steadies the head and prevents you from bumping into the patient's forehead during the examination. If necessary, use the thumb of this hand to gently lift up the patient's eyelid. Instruct the patient to look straight ahead. Aim the beam of light at the pupil from a distance of about 15 inches and slightly lateral to the patient's line of vision. The light beam is on target when the eye appears red-orange (the red reflex); the red-orange color is the light reflecting from the retina. Move straight in toward the patient, never losing the red reflex, until your forehead nearly touches the patient's forehead. Focus by changing diopters (one diopter at a time) until the internal structures of the eye are in clear focus. The back of the eye is curved; any side-to-side, in-and-out, or up-and-down movement changes the focal distance.

Inspect the retinal blood vessels, optic disc, physiologic cup, macula, and retina through the ophthalmoscope (Figure 4-7). No set sequence is followed in visualizing these structures. Inspect the retina, the red-orange area on which the other structures are located, for lesions (Table 4-5). The retinal blood vessels are usually the first structures seen. The retinal arteries and veins emerge from the optic disc and have the highest density in the vicinity of the optic disc. Retinal arteries are thinner and brighter red than retinal veins. Note the size, color, and status of the arteriovenous crossings in all regions of the eyes.

The optic disc, the head of the optic nerve (also known as the *blind spot*), is a yellowish pink ovoid 1.5 mm in diameter with sharp margins (the margins closest to the nose may be blurred). The physiologic cup, the depressed center of the optic disc, is lighter in color than the optic disc and normally occupies about one third of the

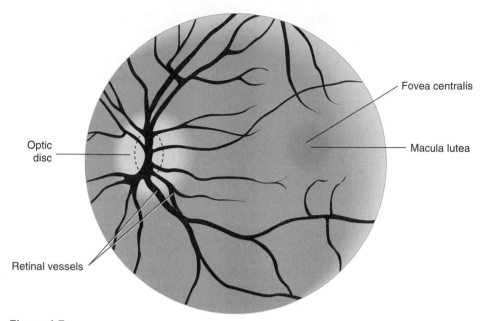

Figure 4-7
Retinal Landmarks.
The retina as seen through the ophthalmoscope. (From Thibodeau GA, Patton KT: *Anatomy & physiology*, ed 9, St Louis, 2003, Mosby.)

diameter of the optic disc (cup-to-disc ratio). Inspect the optic disc for size, shape, and sharpness of the borders and estimate the cup-to-disc ratio.

The macula is a small, round, and extremely light-sensitive area located about two disc-diameters temporally from the optic disc in an area nearly free of retinal blood vessels; the red-free filter is used to inspect the macula. The fovea is the slightly depressed area in the center of the macula.

TERMINOLOGY

acromegaly: A pituitary disorder characterized by a massive face with enlarged lower jaw, prominent nose and eyebrows, and coarse facial features

astigmatism: A condition characterized by unequal curvatures of the cornea

TABLE **4-5**	

Retinal Lesions

Description	Etiology
Red, linear or flame-shaped	Bleeding in nerve fiber retinal layer
Red, round	Bleeding in deeper retinal layers
Black	Retinitis pigmentosus, melanoma, retinal degeneration
White, cotton-wool appearance	Hypertension, diabetes

AV nicking: An abnormality visualized on funduscopic examination and associated with hypertension; at arteriovenous crossings the vein appears to stop abruptly on either side of the arteriole

AV tapering: An abnormality visualized on funduscopic examination and associated with hypertension; at arteriovenous crossings the vein appears to taper off on either side of the arteriole

Bell's palsy: Unilateral paralysis of the facial nerve

Chvostek's sign: Contraction or spasm of the facial muscles associated with tetany and hypocalcemia; elicited by tapping the face sharply with a finger just in front of the external auditory meatus over the facial nerve

conjunctival injection: Dilated conjunctival vessels

copper wires: An abnormality visualized on funduscopic examination and associated with hypertension; a coppery strip of light appears along the surface of the vessel

corneal arcus: A thin, gray-white circle around the cornea; associated with aging

deep hemorrhage: An abnormality visualized on funduscopic examination and associated with diabetes; appears as small, irregular red spots in the retina

exophthalmos: Abnormal protrusion of the eyeball; associated with Graves' disease

fetor hepaticus: A musty odor of breath associated with severe parenchymal liver disease

fissured tongue: Increased tongue fissures; benign; sometimes associated with aging

flame hemorrhage: An abnormality visualized on funduscopic examination; associated with hypertension; appears as small, linear hemorrhages in the retina

geographic tongue: Denuded areas of papillae; benign

hairy tongue: Elongated papillae; benign; associated with antibiotic therapy

hirsutism: Increased hair growth in androgen-sensitive areas (e.g., beard or mustache areas); associated with ovarian, adrenal, thyroid, and pituitary disorders and some medications

hyperopia: Farsightedness

Koplik's spots: Small blue-white spots with red margins found on the mucous membranes near the parotid duct; associated with measles; appear before the skin lesions are visible

microaneurysms: An abnormality visualized on funduscopic examination; associated with diabetes; appear as tiny red spots in the macular area

muddy sclera: Brownish sclera; benign; commonly found in dark-skinned individuals

myopia: Nearsightedness

normocephalic, atraumatic: A physical examination finding meaning that the head is a normal size and shape and no evidence of trauma is present

palpebral fissure: The space, when the eyes are open, between the upper and lower eyelids

periorbital edema: Puffiness of the upper and lower eyelids

Rinne test: A hearing test that compares air and bone conduction

smooth red tongue: Finding associated with deficiencies of vitamin B_{12}, niacin, and iron

Weber's test: A hearing test that compares bone conduction in both ears
xanthelasma: Yellow, raised, well-circumscribed plaques found in the skin
around the eyelids; associated with hypercholesterolemia

CHEST AND LUNGS

Assessment of the chest and lungs requires a clear understanding of pulmonary
anatomy, landmarks, and reference points. The ribs, clavicle, scapula, and vertebrae
serve as useful landmarks. Count ribs on the anterior chest by placing a finger in the
substernal notch and sliding the finger from the substernal notch left or right to the
space between the first and second ribs; count the intercostal spaces or ribs from that
point. On the posterior chest, the spinous process of the seventh cervical vertebra is
quite prominent when the neck is flexed forward. The first thoracic vertebra is just
below the seventh cervical vertebra; count the vertebrae from that point. Vertical reference points include the midsternal, midclavicular, anterior axillary, midaxillary,
posterior axillary, scapular, and vertebral lines (Figure 4-8).

The anterior and posterior positions of the five lobes of the lungs are different
(Figure 4-9). On the anterior chest, the apex of the lung extends 3 to 4 cm above the
medial end of the clavicles. The base of the lung extends to approximately the sixth
to eighth rib. The horizontal fissure separating the right upper and middle lobes is
located from the fourth rib at the midsternal line to the fifth rib at the midaxillary
line. The oblique fissure separating the right middle and lower lobes is located from
the fifth rib at the midaxillary line to the sixth rib at the midclavicular line; the left
oblique fissure separating the left upper and lower lobes is located at a similar position on the left. On the posterior chest, the right and left oblique fissures separating
the right upper and lower lobes and left upper and lower lobes, respectively, are
located from approximately the third thoracic vertebra medially to the sixth rib lat-
erally. The base of the lung extends to approximately the ninth to the twelfth thoracic vertebra.

INSPECTION

Inspect the chest throughout at least one complete inspiratory-expiratory cycle.
Note chest wall abnormalities, accessory muscle use, the anteroposterior diameter,
and skeletal abnormalities.

PERCUSSION

Percuss over intercostal spaces to assess lung density. Percussion over normal lung
tissue creates a loud, low-pitched, resonant note. Percussion over areas of lung with
increased air volume (e.g., emphysema) creates a very loud, low-pitched, hyperreso-
nant note. Areas of consolidation (fluid) produce a dull or flat percussion note; shifting dullness is associated with freely moving fluid within the pleural cavity. Assess all
lobes, comparing the right and left lobes.

Percuss to determine diaphragmatic location and excursion. Determine the location of each diaphragm with the lungs fully expanded and emptied; the difference
between the two positions is the diaphragmatic excursion. Percuss down the posterior chest between the vertebral column and the scapula from about the sixth rib
downward with the lungs fully expanded; repeat with the lungs emptied. The
diaphragm is located where the percussion note changes from resonant to dull.
Normal diaphragmatic excursion is about 3 to 5 cm for females and 5 to 6 cm for
males; the right diaphragm is slightly higher than the left.

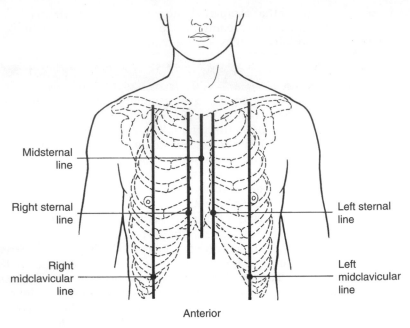

Anterior

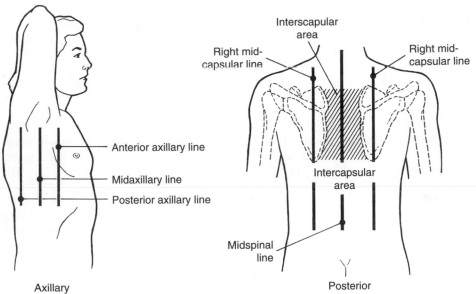

Axillary

Posterior

Figure 4-8
Thorax Topography.
Anterior, posterior, and axillary landmarks. (From Delp MH, Manning RT: *Major's physical diagnosis,* ed 9, Philadelphia, 1991, WB Saunders.)

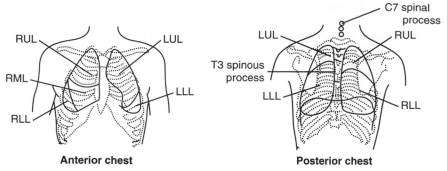

Figure 4-9
Anterior and Posterior Chest Topography.
Anterior lobes (right upper, right middle, right lower, left upper, and left lower lobes) and posterior lobes (right upper, right lower, left upper, and left lower lobes).

PALPATION

Palpate the chest for masses, pulsations, crepitation, and tactile fremitus. To assess for tactile fremitus, place the palm of the hand on the chest and have the patient say "ninety-nine" or "one-two-three."

AUSCULTATION

Auscultate the lungs with a stethoscope. On the posterior chest, auscultate between the scapulae and vertebral column. Place the diaphragm of the stethoscope flat against the chest wall and instruct the patient to breathe deeply and slowly through the mouth each time the stethoscope touches the skin. Assess at least one complete respiratory cycle over each anterior and posterior lobe, comparing right and left sides; assess more thoroughly if abnormalities are detected.

Breath sounds are described as tracheal, bronchial, bronchovesicular, or vesicular. Breath sounds are distinguishable through auscultation over areas of the lungs that normally produce the sounds (i.e., auscultation over the trachea, large central bronchi, small airways just distal to the central bronchi, and small lateral airways identifies tracheal, bronchial, bronchovesicular, and vesicular breath sounds, respectively). These breath sounds are considered abnormal if heard over other areas of the lungs. Other abnormal breath sounds include wheezes, rhonchi, stridor, and crackles. A pleural friction rub, created when the visceral and parietal pleurae rub together, sounds like creaking leather and is heard best at the base of the lung. Voice sounds (egophony, whispered pectoriloquy) are transmitted more clearly over areas of consolidation; vocal resonance is decreased over areas of hyperinflation.

TERMINOLOGY

apnea: Absence of respiration
barrel chest: An anteroposterior diameter ratio of 1:1; associated with diseases characterized by air trapping (e.g., COPD)
Biot's respiration: Irregular respiration; may occur in meningitis
bradypnea: Abnormally slow respiratory rate with regular rhythm and normal depth of breathing; associated with central nervous system depressants and elevated intracranial pressure

bronchial breath sounds: Loud, high-pitched, normal breath sounds heard over the manubrium; normal inspiratory/expiratory ratio of 1:3

bronchovesicular breath sounds: Normal breath sounds heard over the main stem bronchi just distal to the central airways; softer and lower pitched than tracheal breath sounds with equal inspiratory and expiratory duration and pitch

Cheyne-Stokes respiration: A cyclic, abnormal respiratory pattern characterized by a gradual increase in the depth and rate of respiration followed by a gradual decrease in the depth and rate ending in apnea; characteristic of diseases that affect the central respiratory centers

consolidation: Increased density

crackles: Discontinuous, short-duration, bubbling sounds

crepitation: Crackling

dullness or flatness: Soft, medium-pitched percussion notes elicited over areas of increased density

egophony: Altered vocal resonance over areas of consolidation; the spoken "e-e-e-e" is transmitted as "a-a-a-a"

eupnea: Normal respiration

funnel chest (pectus excavatum):   Finding in which the lower part of the sternum is depressed

hyperpnea: Increased depth and rate of respiration

hyperresonance: A loud, low-pitched percussion note elicited over areas of increased air volume

Kussmaul's breathing: Deep, rapid respiration; characteristic of coma and diabetic ketoacidosis

kyphoscoliosis: Combined kyphosis and scoliosis

kyphosis: Abnormal curvature of the spine with backward convexity

pigeon chest: Anterior displacement of the sternum

pleural friction rub: abnormal, creaking leatherlike sound produced when the inflamed surfaces of the visceral and parietal pleura rub against one another

resonance: The loud, low-pitched percussion note elicited over normal lung tissue

rhonchi: Coarse, rattling, abnormal breath sounds; often change location after coughing

scoliosis: Abnormal lateral curvature of the spine

stridor: Abnormal, high-pitched, continuous lung sounds heard over the upper airway

tachypnea: Increased respiratory rate

tactile fremitus: Palpable vocal vibrations felt through the chest wall; increased over areas of consolidation; decreased over obstructed areas and pleural abnormalities

tracheal breath sounds: Very loud and high-pitched harsh normal breath sounds heard over the extrathoracic trachea

tracheobronchial breath sounds: Loud, high-pitched, normal breath sounds heard over large bronchi; a slight pause occurs between inspiratory and expiratory sounds; inspiratory duration shorter than expiratory duration

tympany: Loud, drumlike percussion notes elicited over hyperinflated areas

vesicular breath sounds: Soft, low-pitched, normal breath sounds heard over peripheral lung tissue; inspiratory duration longer than expiratory duration

wheezes: Abnormal, high-pitched, continuous breath sounds; associated with airway obstruction

whispered pectoriloquy: Whispered voice sounds are transmitted more loudly and clearly than normal; associated with areas of cavitation and consolidation

CARDIOVASCULAR SYSTEM

Assessment of the cardiovascular system requires a clear understanding of cardiac anatomy, landmarks, and reference points (Figure 4-10). The right ventricle occupies most of the anterior cardiac surface; the right atrium occupies a narrow border from the third to the fifth rib just right of the sternum. The other chambers of the heart are normally too posterior to be identified on examination. The left ventricular apex (apical impulse or point of maximal impulse) is normally located at the intersection of the fifth intercostal space and the midclavicular line. The base of the heart is located between the right second intercostal space medial to the sternum to the left second intercostal space medial to the sternum.

The techniques of inspection, palpation, and auscultation are used to assess the heart. By convention, the examination is conducted from the patient's right side. Although very light percussion may be used to determine the cardiac borders and assess for the presence of pericardial effusions, aortic aneurysm, and mediastinal tumors, percussion is not a part of the routine cardiovascular examination.

INSPECTION
Inspect the chest for visible cardiac motions. Estimate the jugular venous pressure (JVP) and assess the jugular venous waveforms by observing pulsations in the jugular vein with the patient supine and the head of the bed elevated to 15 to 30 degrees. The jugular vein is located in the neck next to the point where the sternocleidomastoid muscle attaches to the clavicle. The JVP is the vertical distance between the highest point at which pulsations of the jugular vein can be seen and the sternal angle. Because JVP depends on the angle of elevation of the head, record both the vertical distance and the angle of elevation. However, estimation of JVP by this method is highly inaccurate. More generally, the right atrial pressure is high (>15 mm Hg) if the jugular vein is distended to the jaw when the patient is seated at a 90-degree angle. The jugular venous waveforms (Figure 4-11) are easiest to see in the right jugular vein, which is straighter than the left. The *a* wave results from atrial contraction. The *v* wave results from the pressures transmitted just before the opening of the tricuspid valve. The *x* descent follows the *a* wave and represents decreased pressure as blood flows into the atrium. The *y* descent follows the *v* wave and represents decreased pressure as blood flows into the ventricle. Normally only the *a* and *v* waves are visible.

PALPATION
Palpate for the point of maximal impulse (PMI), local and general cardiac motion, and cardiac thrills. The PMI normally has a diameter of about 2 cm and is located within about 10 cm of the midsternal line; use the fingertips to locate the PMI. The PMI is easier to identify if the patient sits up and leans forward than if the patient is supine. Palpate for local and general cardiac motion with the fingertips with the patient in a supine position. Pericardial friction rubs and thrills may be palpable.

Palpate for the radial, carotid, brachial, femoral, popliteal, posterior tibial, and dorsalis pedis peripheral pulses (Figure 4-12). Rate the strength of the pulse as

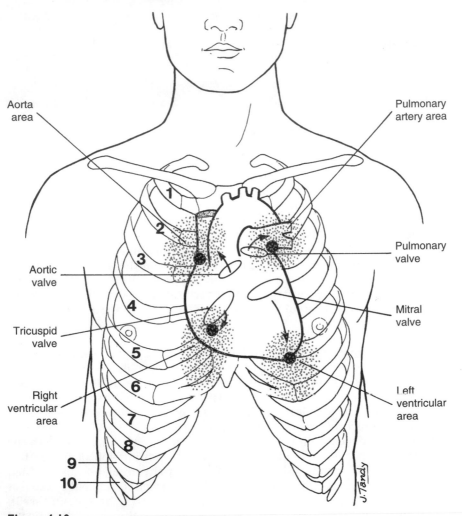

Figure 4-10
Cardiovascular Topography.
Cardiovascular landmarks and auscultatory areas. (From Delp MH, Manning RT: *Major's physical diagnosis*, ed 9, Philadelphia, 1991, WB Saunders.)

normal, diminished, or absent; a rating scale may be used. The typical rating scale is a 0 to 4+ scale, with 2+ denoting a normal strength pulse (Table 4-6). Palpate the radial artery for heart rate and cardiac rhythm.

AUSCULTATION
Auscultate the heart with a stethoscope. Use the diaphragm to assess higher-pitched sounds (e.g., S_1, S_2, S_3, S_4); apply the diaphragm tightly to the skin. Use the bell to assess lower-pitched sounds (e.g., murmurs); apply the bell loosely to the skin. A great deal of practice and experience is required to identify and distinguish among the variety of normal and abnormal heart sounds. Heart sounds are very soft; it may help to listen in a quiet area or to close the eyes to reduce conflicting stimuli.

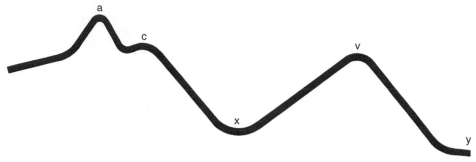

Figure 4-11
Jugular Venous Waveforms.
The jugular venous waveforms vary with atrial pressures. *a*, Atrial contraction; *c*, bulging of tricuspid valve into the right atrium; *x*, decreased pressures as blood flows into the atrium; *v*, pressure increased just before tricuspid valve opens; *y*, decreased pressure as blood flows into the ventricle.

The four auscultatory areas are identified in Figure 4-8. The auscultatory areas are close to, but not the same as, the anatomic locations of the valves. The aortic auscultatory area is located over the second intercostal space at the right sternal border, the pulmonic auscultatory area is located over the second intercostal space at the left sternal border, the tricuspid auscultatory area is located over the left lower sternal border, and the mitral auscultatory area is located at the cardiac apex (fifth intercostal space midclavicular line).

The first heart sound (S_1), created by mitral and tricuspid valve closure, is loudest at the cardiac apex. The second heart sound (S_2), created by aortic and pulmonic valve closure, is loudest at the base of the heart. The second heart sound can be "split" into distinct aortic and pulmonic components by deep inspiration (physiologic splitting) or disease (e.g., pulmonary hypertension). The third heart sound (S_3), an abnormal heart sound associated with volume overload, is a soft sound heard just after S_2. The fourth heart sound (S_4), an abnormal heart sound associated with pressure overload, is a soft sound heard just before S_1. S_1 and S_2 are assessed in all four auscultatory areas with the patient in the upright and supine positions. Note the relationship of breathing to the intensity of the cardiac sounds. Palpate the carotid artery to help determine the timing of cardiac events and sounds (the S_1 precedes and the S_2 follows the carotid pulse).

Other abnormal heart sounds include opening snaps (associated with mitral stenosis), ejection clicks (associated with sudden dilation of the aorta and the pulmonary artery), and midsystolic clicks (associated with floppy mitral valves). Gallops are exaggerated normal diastolic sounds; friction rubs are associated with pericarditis. Some heart sounds are heard best if the patient is in a specific body position. For example, aortic sounds and pericardial friction rubs are heard best when the patient sits up and leans forward. S_3, S_4, and aortic insufficiency and mitral stenosis murmurs are heard best when the patient is supine and turned to the left.

Murmurs (abnormal heart sounds created by turbulent flow across a valve or the septum and by diseases such as anemia and hyperthyroidism) are described according to their timing in the cardiac cycle (systolic murmurs occur between S_1 and S_2; diastolic murmurs occur between S_2 and S_1), loudest location, radiation, shape (crescendo, decrescendo, crescendo-decrescendo, continuous), duration (continuous; early, mid, late systolic; diastolic; holosystolic; pansystolic), intensity (grade I

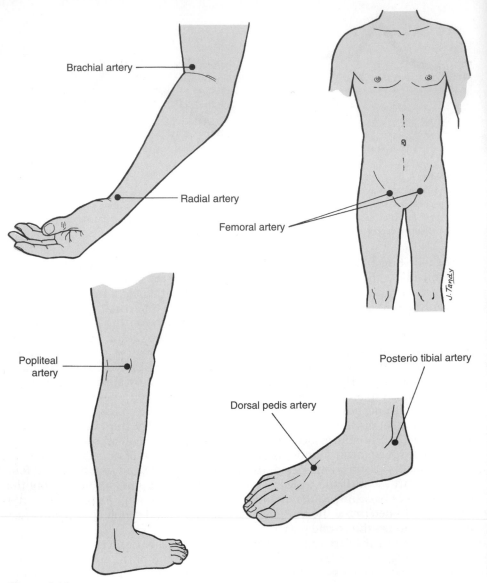

Figure 4-12
Peripheral Pulses.
The peripheral pulses are located over major arteries in the upper extremities, inguinal area, and lower extremities.

through VI) (Table 4-7), and pitch or quality of sound (low, medium, high). A palpable murmur is known as a *thrill*.

Auscultation also is used to detect vascular murmurs, known as *bruits*. Bruits (sounds made by turbulent blood flow) are heard over vessels with constricted lumens. The carotid and femoral arteries are routinely assessed for bruits; bruits are sometimes found over the vertebral, subclavian, and abdominal arteries.

TABLE 4-6

Peripheral Vascular Pulse Rating Scale

Rating	Meaning
0	No pulse palpable
1+	Markedly impaired pulse
2+	Normal pulse
3+	Increased pulse
4+	Bounding (markedly increased) pulse

BLOOD PRESSURE

The peripheral blood pressure is measured with a stethoscope, blood pressure cuff, and mercury or aneroid sphygmomanometer. Both types of sphygmomanometers are accurate and easy to use; however, the mercury column must be kept vertical and the meniscus read at eye level. Aneroid sphygmomanometers must be recalibrated periodically.

Use an appropriately sized cuff. Cuffs that are too short or too narrow falsely elevate the blood pressure. The cuff width should be about 40% of the limb circumference, and the cuff length should be about 80% of the limb circumference. Position the cuff correctly. Place the arterial portion of the cuff directly over the brachial artery with the bottom of the edge approximately 2.5 cm above the antecubital crease (Figure 4-13); palpate for the brachial artery before positioning the cuff on the arm. Support the patient's arm at the level of the heart; tensed muscles falsely elevate the blood pressure. Place the stethoscope over the brachial artery and inflate the cuff to about 20 to 30 mm Hg over the predicted systolic blood pressure. Deflate the cuff slowly (approximately 3 mm Hg per second). There are no audible sounds (Korotkoff sounds) until the cuff pressure approximates the systolic blood pressure; the systolic blood pressure is the pressure at which at least two Korotkoff sounds are audible. As the pressure falls, the sounds become louder and then slowly diminish before disappearing altogether. The diastolic pressure is the pressure at which the beats are no longer audible. Depending on the clinical situation, it may be necessary

TABLE 4-7

Murmur Rating Scale

Grade	Meaning
I	Very faint
II	Soft
III	Moderately loud
IV	Loud
V	Very loud; may be heard with the stethoscope partially off the chest wall
VI	Very loud; can be heard with the stethoscope off the chest wall

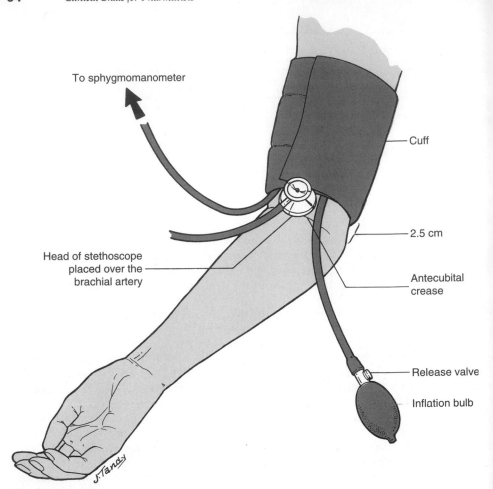

To sphygmomanometer

Cuff

2.5 cm

Head of stethoscope
placed over the
brachial artery

Antecubital
crease

Release valve

Inflation bulb

Figure 4-13
Blood Pressure Cuff Position.
The blood pressure cuff and stethoscope must be positioned correctly to obtain an accurate assessment of
the blood pressure.

to obtain the blood pressure in both arms or in more than one body position (i.e., sitting and standing, sitting and supine). Do not reinflate the cuff after partial deflation; cuff reinflation causes venous congestion and inaccurate blood pressure assessments.

TERMINOLOGY
    bradycardia: A slow (<50 beats per minute) heart rate
    bruit: An abnormal auscultatory sound heard over a blood vessel; associated with turbulent blood flow
    crescendo, decrescendo murmur: A murmur that increases and then decreases in intensity

diastolic murmur: A murmur heard during diastole

ejection clicks: Abnormal heart sounds caused by dilation of the aortic and pulmonary arteries

gallop rhythms: Exaggerated diastolic heart sounds

holosystolic murmur: A murmur heard throughout systole

hypertension: Elevated blood pressure

hypotension: Low blood pressure

midsystolic clicks: Abnormal heart sounds caused by floppy mitral valves

opening snap: An abnormal diastolic heart sound caused by the opening of a stenotic mitral valve

orthostatic hypotension: A fall in systolic blood pressure of 15 mm Hg or more when the patient assumes a more upright position

pansystolic murmur: A murmur heard throughout systole

pericardial friction rub: An abnormal sound created when the visceral and parietal pericardial membranes rub against one another

point of maximal impulse (PMI):   Right ventricular thrust (apical impulse)

pulsus alternans: Regular alteration of high and low pulse beats; associated with heart failure

pulsus paradoxus: Decreased systolic blood pressure with inspiration; normally about 5 mm Hg

regurgitant murmur: A murmur produced by backflow of blood across an incompetent valve

S_1:   The first heart sound; produced by mitral and tricuspid valve closure

S_2:   The second heart sound; produced by aortic and pulmonic valve closure

S_3:   The third heart sound; produced by the sudden distention of the ventricular wall during ventricular filling; associated with heart failure

S_4:   The fourth heart sound; produced by increased left ventricular end-diastolic pressure and loss of ventricular distensibility; associated with hypertension

split S_2:   Finding in which both components of the second heart sound (aortic and pulmonic) are distinguishable; may result from deep inspiration and any disease that delays the closure of the pulmonic valve

stenosis murmur: A murmur produced by the pathologic narrowing of the orifice of a valve

systolic ejection murmur: A murmur caused by increased flow across a normal valve, valvular or subvalvular stenosis, or other deformity of the valve

systolic murmur: A murmur heard during systole

tachycardia: A rapid (>100 beats per minute) heart rate

thrill: Palpable vibrations produced by turbulent blood flow

BREASTS AND AXILLAE

Inspect and palpate the breasts and axillae.

INSPECTION

Inspect the breasts with the patient in sitting and supine positions. Inspect for size, symmetry, contour, and appearance of the skin. Abnormal findings on inspection include visible masses, dimpling, localized flattening, rashes, ulcers, and discharge from the nipple.

PALPATION

Palpate the breasts for nodules, indurations, and areas of tenderness or increased warmth. The axillary lymph nodes, including the pectoral, subscapular, and lateral groups, are located high in the axilla close to the ribs. Palpate the nodes for size, consistency, and tenderness.

TERMINOLOGY

gynecomastia: Hypertrophy of breast tissue; associated with liver cirrhosis, Addison's disease, Klinefelter's syndrome, and some medications (e.g., spironolactone)

mastodynia: Painful breasts

peau d'orange: Breast skin with an orange-peel appearance (prominent pores); indicates lymphatic obstruction and is an important sign of malignancy

retraction: Dimpling of the skin, nipple retraction or inversion

ABDOMEN

The abdomen is evaluated through inspection, percussion, palpation, and auscultation. Auscultation must be performed immediately after inspection to avoid acute examination-related changes in abdominal sounds. The examination is conducted at the patient's right side with the patient lying supine. Instruct the patient to bend the knees and place the feet flat on the examining table if the abdomen is tense. To decrease the sensitivity of ticklish patients, have them place their hand over your hand.

Assessment of the abdomen requires a clear understanding of abdominal anatomy (Table 4-8), landmarks, and reference points. The abdominal area is divided into four quadrants (right upper, right lower, left upper, left lower) by imaginary vertical and horizontal lines that cross at the umbilicus (Figure 4-14); report findings by quadrant (e.g., right upper quadrant tenderness).

INSPECTION

Inspect the abdomen for the appearance of the skin, umbilicus, and abdominal contour (scaphoid, protuberant); note visible aortic and hepatic pulsations, peristaltic waves, and fluid shifts. Free fluid in the peritoneal cavity may shift with position, causing bulging at the flanks when the patient is supine.

AUSCULTATION

Auscultate the abdomen for bowel sounds and abdominal bruits. Bowel sounds, produced by the movement of fluid and air in the bowel, vary from low rumbles in loosely stretched intestines to high-pitched tinkling sounds in tightly stretched intestines. Bowel sounds audible without a stethoscope are called *borborygmi*. Normal peristaltic movement creates normal bowel sounds; bowel sounds are absent if there is no peristalsis. Normal bowel sounds occur approximately every 10 seconds. Auscultate for 2 minutes if normal bowel sounds are present and for 3 minutes if bowel sounds are absent. Listen in one quadrant to screen for bowel sounds. Depending of the clinical situation, it may be necessary to listen for bowel sounds in all four quadrants. Listen for bruits over the aorta, right and left renal arteries, right and left iliac arteries, and right and left femoral arteries; friction rubs may be heard over the liver and spleen.

TABLE **4-8**

Abdominal Anatomy

Quadrant	Structure
Right upper quadrant	Liver, gallbladder, a portion of the ascending colon, a portion of the transverse colon, pylorus, duodenum,* head of pancreas,* right adrenal gland,* upper pole of the right kidney*
Right lower quadrant	Appendix, cecum, portion of the ascending colon, right ureter, lower pole of right kidney,* bladder (if enlarged), right ovary, right fallopian tube, uterus (if enlarged), right spermatic cord
Left upper quadrant	Liver, spleen, stomach, body of pancreas,* portion of transverse colon, portion of descending colon, left adrenal gland*
Left lower quadrant	Sigmoid colon, portion of descending colon, lower pole of left kidney,* left ureter, bladder (if enlarged), left ovary, left fallopian tube, uterus (if enlarged), left spermatic cord

*Normally too deep to be palpable.

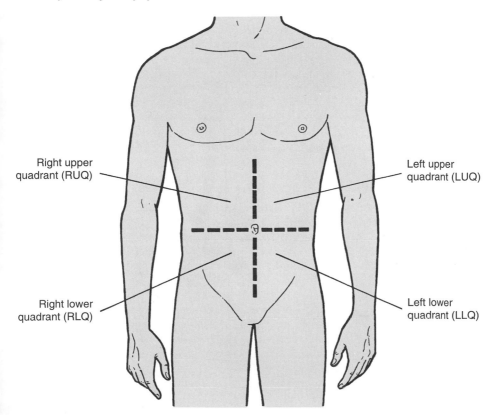

Right upper quadrant (RUQ)

Left upper quadrant (LUQ)

Right lower quadrant (RLQ)

Left lower quadrant (LLQ)

Figure 4-14
Abdominal Quadrants.
The abdomen is divided into four quadrants (right upper, right lower, left upper, and left lower quadrants).

PERCUSSION

Percuss to determine the liver span and to differentiate between abdominal fluid and air. Percussion over the liver produces a dull note; percussion over air-filled loops of bowel produces a hollow tympanic note. The normal liver span along the right mid-clavicular line is about 10 cm. Determine the liver span by percussing down the right midclavicular line starting at midchest (Figure 4-15). The liver span is evident as the percussion note changes from the resonant lung note to a dull liver note to a tympanic colonic note.

Percuss each quadrant. Shifting dullness indicates freely moving fluid. Air-filled loops of bowel float to the surface of the abdomen and may obscure abdominal fluid. In these cases a puddle sign is elicited by having the patient lie supine on the abdomen for a few moments and then shift to a hands-and-knees position. The fluid

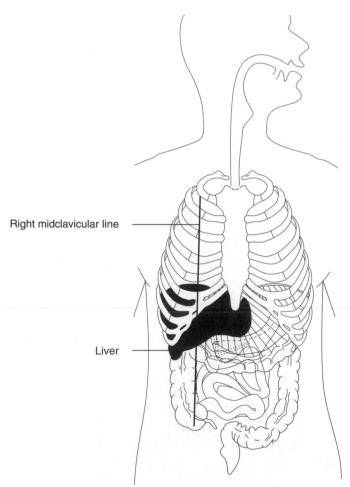

Right midclavicular line

Liver

Figure 4-15
Liver Span.
The liver span is percussed in the right midclavicular line.

collects, or puddles, over the gravity-dependent portion of the abdomen and can be identified with percussion.

PALPATION

Palpate tender or rigid areas with light palpation; use the pads of the fingertips with light pressure (as if kneading bread dough). Use deep palpation (significant downward pressure) to determine the outlines of the abdominal organs and to assess the size, shape, mobility, and tenderness of the lymph nodes. Palpate all four quadrants.

Palpate for the liver edge using deep palpation just below the right costal margin during full inspiration. Place the left hand under the back on the posterior twelfth rib along the iliac crest. Place the right hand in the right upper quadrant parallel and lateral to the rectus muscle and a couple of inches below the lower margin of dullness as identified on percussion. Instruct the patient to take a deep breath and hold the breath. Lift the left hand upward and push the right hand inward and upward as the patient inspires. The liver edge, normally smooth, firm, and regular, slides over the fingertips as the liver is pushed downward by the expanding lungs.

The kidneys may be palpable on deep palpation, but the normal-sized spleen, duodenum, and pancreas cannot be palpated. The tip of an enlarged spleen may be palpated near the left tenth rib just posterior to the midaxillary line. Intraabdominal structures may not be palpable if the abdomen is obese or distended by fluid. Abdominal rigidity (tensing of the abdominal muscles) may be present if the abdomen is tender. Rebound tenderness (tenderness when deep pressure is released) may be elicited if the parietal peritoneum is inflamed.

A fluid wave may be elicited in patients with abdominal ascites. Generate a fluid wave by pressing the ulnar surface of one hand midline against the surface of the abdomen; this dampens the transmission of the wave through the fat layer. Then sharply tap the lateral wall of the abdomen with the other hand. The fluid wave is transmitted to the other side of the abdomen and felt by the hand placed on the opposite lateral abdominal wall.

TERMINOLOGY

ascites: Free fluid in the peritoneal cavity

borborygmi: Very loud gurgling and tinkling bowel sounds audible without a stethoscope; associated with hyperperistalsis

caput medusa: Dilated veins radiating from the umbilicus; associated with portal vein obstruction

costal margin: The edge of the lower rib cage

costovertebral angle: The angle formed by the intersection of the rib cage and the vertebral column

epigastric region: The upper central abdominal area

fluid wave: Associated with free fluid in the abdominal cavity

hypogastric region: The lower central abdominal area

peristalsis: The circular intestinal contractions that propel the intestinal contents forward

puddle sign: Gravity-dependent pooling of fluid at the surface of the abdomen

rebound tenderness: Pain elicited when abdominal hand pressure is abruptly removed; associated with parietal peritoneal membrane inflammation

Rovsing's sign: Right lower quadrant pain elicited by left-sided abdominal pressure; associated with appendicitis

scaphoid: Concave-appearing abdomen

shifting dullness: Dull percussion notes that shift as the patient shifts position; associated with free fluid in the abdominal cavity

spider telangiectasia (spider angioma):   Dilated small surface arteries that appear as small red spots with multiple radiating arms; associated with portal hypertension

striae: Discolored stripes of skin that result from ruptured elastic fibers; striae are pinkish or bluish when relatively new and more whitish when older

suprapubic region: The abdominal area just above the pubic arch

umbilical region: The area around the umbilicus

GENITOURINARY SYSTEM

The genitourinary system is evaluated using inspection and palpation.

INSPECTION

Inspect sacrococcygeal and perianal areas for lumps, ulcerations, rashes, swelling, external hemorrhoids, and excoriations. Inspect the female external genitalia (mons pubis, labia, perineum, labia minora, clitoris, urethral orifice, and introitus) for abnormalities, including lumps, ulcerations, rashes, swelling, excoriations, and discharge. Inspect the male external genitalia (penis and scrotum) for contour and abnormalities, including lumps, ulcerations, inflammation, excoriations, and swelling.

The female pelvic examination consists of an inspection and palpation (see later discussion). Inspect the vaginal wall and cervix for color, lesions, and the shape of the cervix and cervical os. Note the position of the cervix. Cervical cells may be collected for cytologic evaluation (the Papanicolaou [Pap] smear).

PALPATION

Palpate the anus and rectal wall for tone and tenderness. The prostate is palpated for size, consistency, and tenderness. Palpate the penis for indurations or other abnormalities and palpate the scrotal structures (testis and epididymis) for size, shape, consistency, and tenderness. Palpate the inguinal and femoral areas for bulges that may indicate hernias.

Palpate the uterus and ovaries for size, shape, consistency, masses, tenderness, and mobility. The bimanual examination is performed by palpating the internal structures between a hand placed on the abdominal wall and a finger placed in the vagina. The combined rectovaginal examination is performed by palpating the adnexa, cul-de-sac, and uterosacral ligaments between a finger placed in the vagina and a finger placed in the rectum.

TERMINOLOGY

angiokeratoma: Red, slightly raised, pinpoint benign scrotal lesions; common after age 50 years

anteverted, anteflexed uterus: Normal uterine position

chancre: A hard infectious venereal ulcer

chancroid: A soft infectious venereal ulcer

condylomata acuminatum: Venereal warts

gravid: Pregnant

hernia: Protrusion of an organ through the muscular wall that normally contains the organ

hydrocele: Serous fluid–containing cavity
Papanicolaou (Pap) smear: Screening technique for cervical carcinoma
prostatic hypertrophy: Enlarged prostate
varicocele: Enlarged spermatic cord

MUSCULOSKELETAL SYSTEM

The musculoskeletal system is evaluated primarily through inspection and palpation.

INSPECTION
Inspect the musculoskeletal system for symmetry, proportion, and muscular development; note the curvature of the spine. Observe the gait; stance; and ability to stand, sit, rise from a sitting position, and grasp objects. Inspect the muscles for symmetry.

PALPATION
Palpate the large and small joints. Assess joint range of motion. Decreased range of motion is associated with arthritis, fibrosis in or around the joint, tissue inflammation around the joint, and fixed (immobile) joints. Increased range of motion indicates increased joint mobility and may be a sign of joint instability. Limits or extension of the range of motion of a joint are reported in degrees. Assess joint tenderness by gently palpating in and around the joint. Assess the areas in and around the joints for abnormalities such as warmth, tenderness, crepitation, and deformities.

TERMINOLOGY
activities of daily living (ADLs):   Routine activities such as getting dressed, cleaning the teeth, combing or brushing the hair, bathing, and feeding oneself
boutonniere deformity: Flexion of the proximal interphalangeal joint with hyperextension of the distal interphalangeal joint
crepitation: Audible or palpable crackling sounds
dorsiflexion: Inward flexion
eversion: The turning of the toes onto the great toe (foot flexed outward)
extension: The bending of a joint to bring the joint parallel to the long axis
flexion: The bending of a joint to bring the parts of the joint into close approximation
gait: The way a person walks
inversion: The turning of the toes onto the small toes (foot flexed inward)
kyphosis: Convex backward spinal curvature
list: Lateral deviation of the spine
lordosis: Anteroposterior curvature of the spine (i.e., an accentuation of the normal lumbar curve)
neutral range of motion: Zero degrees
plantar flexion: Downward flexion of the foot
radial deviation: Deviation of the fingers toward the radial bone
rheumatoid nodules: Firm, nontender, unattached subcutaneous nodules at pressure points on the extensor surface of the ulna; associated with rheumatoid arthritis
scoliosis: Lateral curvature of the spine

station: The way a person stands
ulnar deviation: Deviation of the fingers toward the ulnar bone

NEUROLOGIC SYSTEM

The neurologic examination assesses mental status, cranial nerve function, sensory and motor function, cerebellar function, and reflexes. Test each component separately; the standard IPPA approach is not used. A complete neurologic assessment is complex and time-consuming; however, unless neurologic abnormalities are suspected or detected, the neurologic examination is limited to a simple screening examination of mental status, major reflexes, and major motor function.

MENTAL STATUS
The standard mental status examination assesses the 12 components listed here. The Mini-Mental Status Examination (MMSE), an abbreviated mental status examination, assesses orientation, speech and vocabulary, memory, calculation, and constructional praxis.

Alertness.   Determine the patient's level of consciousness (awake, alert, confused, unresponsive).

Orientation.   Determine the patient's orientation to person, place, and time. Ask "What is your name?" "Where are you?" and "What is today's date?" (or day, month, year, or season, depending on the patient's circumstances).

Affect.   Determine whether the patient's affect (emotion or mood) is appropriate to the situation.

Speech and Vocabulary.   Have the patient say "no ifs, ands, or buts." Note the patient's vocabulary throughout the interview. Ask the patient to define a series of increasingly difficult words.

Memory (Immediate, Short-Term, and Long-Term Memory).   To assess immediate memory, say a list of single-digit numbers and have the patient immediately repeat the list. To assess short-term memory, have the patient memorize three unrelated words (e.g., cat, bus, pencil). Ask the patient to repeat the words to ensure that the patient knows the words; then ask the patient to repeat the three words a few minutes later. To assess long-term memory, ask the patient about an age-appropriate, well-known historical event (e.g., D-day, the assassination of President Kennedy, the September 11, 2001, attacks).

Judgment.   Ask the patient to interpret a simple problem that involves judgment, such as "What would you do if you noticed a stamped, addressed envelope on the sidewalk near a mailbox?"

Abstract Thinking.   Ask the patient to interpret a common proverb, such as "A bird in hand is worth two in the bush" or "The grass is always greener on the other side of the fence." Alternatively, ask the patient to explain how items are similar or dissimilar (e.g., "What do bananas, apples, and oranges have in common?" or "What is the difference between a book and a videotape?").

Calculation.   Ask the patient to perform serial seven subtractions, starting from 100 (i.e., 100 minus 7 is 93, 93 minus 7 is 86, 86 minus 7 is 79). Alternatively, ask the patient to spell "world" backward.

Object Recognition.   Ask the patient to identify several well-known objects (e.g., watch, belt, ring, coin).

Praxis.   Ask the patient to perform a multistep motor activity (e.g., "Pick up a piece of paper with your left hand, crumple it, and hand it to me").

CRANIAL NERVES
Each of the 12 cranial nerves (Table 4-9) is assessed individually.

I—Olfactory Nerve.   Evaluate the olfactory nerve only if the patient complains of loss of the sense of smell or if the patient has a head injury. Ask the patient to close his or her eyes and identify (one nostril at a time) a familiar odor (e.g., soap, coffee, toothpaste).

II—Optic Nerve.   Test the patient's visual fields (refer to page 72) and ability to discriminate between colors.

III, IV, and VI—Oculomotor, Trochlear, and Abducens Nerves.   Evaluate the oculomotor, trochlear, and abducens nerves (known collectively as the *ocular nerves*) as a

---

TABLE **4-9**

The Cranial Nerves

Cranial Nerve	Function
I—Olfactory	Sense of smell
II—Optic	Vision
III—Oculomotor	Pupillary constriction; upper eyelid elevation; most extraocular movement
IV—Trochlear	Downward and inward eye movements
V—Trigeminal	Temporal and masseter muscles; lateral movement of the jaw
VI—Abducens	Lateral deviation of the eye
VII—Facial	Facial muscle movements; sense of taste on anterior two thirds of the tongue
VIII—Acoustic	Hearing and balance
IX—Glossopharyngeal	Sensation of the posterior position of the eardrum, ear canal, pharynx, and posterior tongue, including taste; motor activity of the pharynx
X—Vagus	Sensation of the pharynx and larynx; motor function of the palate, pharynx, and larynx
XI—Accessory	Motor function of the sternomastoid and upper portion of the trapezius muscle
XII—Hypoglossal	Motor activity of the tongue

group. Observe the size and shape of the pupils, pupillary reaction to light and accommodation, and extraocular movements (refer to page 73).

V—Trigeminal Nerve.   Ask the patient to clench the teeth. Test the patient's ability to sense stimuli (sharp, dull, hot, and cold) over the front half of the head.

VII—Facial Nerve.   To assess motor function, observe facial movements when the patient frowns, smiles, puffs out the cheeks, whistles, and raises the eyebrows. To assess sensory function, test the patient's ability to identify sweet, sour, and salty solutions placed on the sides of the tongue.

VIII—Acoustic Nerve.   Test hearing (see pages 71-72) and balance.

IX and X—Glossopharyngeal and Vagus Nerves.   Assess quality of speech and the gag reflex. Observe the movement of the soft palate and uvula as the patient says "ahh."

XI—Accessory Nerve.   Test the patient's ability to shrug his or her shoulders and turn the chin from side to side against resistance.

XII—Hypoglossal Nerve.   Ask the patient to stick out his or her tongue. Note abnormalities such as fasciculations, asymmetry, deviations, or atrophy.

SENSORY AND MOTOR FUNCTION
Assess sensory function by testing the patient's ability to detect a variety of sensory stimuli. Ask the patient to close his or her eyes. Start distally and work proximally, comparing left and right sides. Ask the patient to identify when and where he or she is touched. Use a variety of stimuli, including light touch (use a wisp of gauze or tissue), pain (use a sharp object such as the broken end of a tongue depressor), and vibration (place a vibrating tuning fork over a bony prominence). A thorough examination tests all major peripheral nerves and dermatomes. Assess tactile localization, proprioception, and discriminative sensations such as two-point discrimination, stereognosis, graphesthesia, and point localization.

Observe the patient for abnormal involuntary muscle movements, resting muscle tone, and strength against resistance. Muscle strength is evaluated using a plus scale, with 0 representing no muscle contraction (complete paralysis) and 5 representing normal muscle strength (Table 4-10). Evaluate motor function by assessing muscle

TABLE 4-10

Muscle Strength Rating Scale

Scale	Meaning
0	No muscle contractility (complete paralysis)
1+	Barely detectable muscle contractility
2+	Active muscle contractility; unable to work against gravity
3+	Active muscle contractility; able to work against gravity but not against resistance
4+	Active muscle contractility; able to work against gravity and some resistance
5+	Active muscle contractility; able to work against gravity and full resistance (normal)

tone during passive flexion and extension (increased resistance, normal, decreased resistance), abduction and adduction, and flexion and extension (Figure 4-16). A thorough examination tests all muscle groups in both the upper and lower extremities.

CEREBELLAR FUNCTION
The finger-to-nose test, heel-to-shin test, rapid alternating movements (e.g., pronation and supination; see Figure 4-16), Romberg test, and gait are used to assess cerebellar function. For the finger-to-nose test hold your finger about an arm's length in front of the patient; ask the patient to quickly and repeatedly touch his or her nose and then your finger. For the heel-to-shin test, instruct the patient to rub the heel down the shin of the opposite leg. The rapid alternating movements test is performed by asking the patient to pronate and supinate the hands rapidly and repeatedly. The Romberg test is performed by instructing the patient to stand with the feet together, arms extended with palms up, and eyes closed. Patients with normal posterior column function maintain the position without moving their feet for balance. Ask the patient to walk straight ahead, turn, return walking on tiptoes, turn, walk away on the heels, turn, and return walking heel-to-toe; observe the gait.

REFLEXES
Assess the physiologic and pathologic reflexes. Ask the patient to relax the area being tested. Test the deep tendon reflexes by striking the tendon briskly with the reflex hammer; the pointed end of the triangular head is generally used. Test the superficial reflexes by gently tapping or stroking the area. Report the results using a plus scale (Table 4-11), with 0 representing complete absence of the reflex, 2+ representing a normal response, and 4+ representing marked hyperreactivity. Reflex test results are often documented using a stick figure representation (Figure 4-17).

Each physiologic reflex tests a different level of spinal cord function. The deep tendon (stretch) reflexes routinely tested include the biceps reflex (C5 and C6), the triceps reflex (C6 to C8), the brachioradialis reflex (C5 and C6), the patellar reflex (L2 to L4), and the Achilles reflex (S1 and S2). The abdominal reflex is a commonly tested superficial reflex. The abdominal reflex is tested by stroking each side of the abdomen above the level of the umbilicus (T8 to T10) and below the level of the umbilicus (T10 to T12); the muscles normally reflexively tighten. The plantar reflex is tested by stroking the lateral aspect of the sole of the foot from the heel to the ball of the foot with a moderately sharp object, such as the handle of the reflex hammer; normally, the toes curl downward.

A variety of pathologic reflexes indicate specific neurologic dysfunction (Table 4-12). An abnormal plantar reflex, known as *Babinski's reflex* or *sign* and indicative of upper motor neuron disease, is characterized by dorsiflexion of the great toe and spreading of the other four toes. The snout, grasp, and sucking reflexes are normally present in infancy but indicate neurologic abnormalities after infancy. Elicit the snout reflex by gently tapping the patient's face just above or below the lips; a positive response is characterized by puckering of the lips. Elicit the grasp reflex by gently stroking the palm of the patient's hand between the thumb and fingers; a positive response is characterized by flexion of the fingers. Elicit the sucking reflex by gently stroking the patient's lips from side to center with a tongue depressor; a positive response is indicated by sucking movements. Elicit the Hoffmann's reflex by dorsiflexing the patient's wrist with the fingers flexed and flicking the middle finger; a positive response is characterized by adduction of the thumb or index finger. The

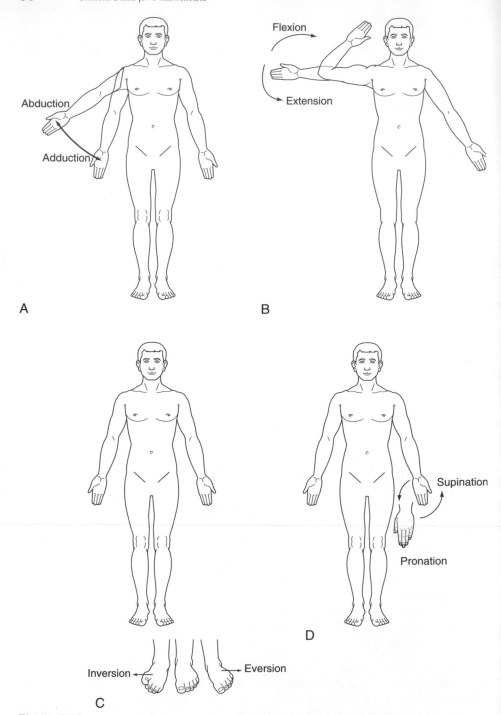

Figure 4-16
Motor Function.
A, Abduction and adduction. **B,** Flexion and extension. **C,** Inversion and eversion. **D,** Pronation and supination.

TABLE 4-11

Reflex Rating Scale

Scale	Meaning
0	No response
1+	Diminished response
2+	Normal physiologic response
3+	Increased response
4+	Hyperreactive; often associated with clonus

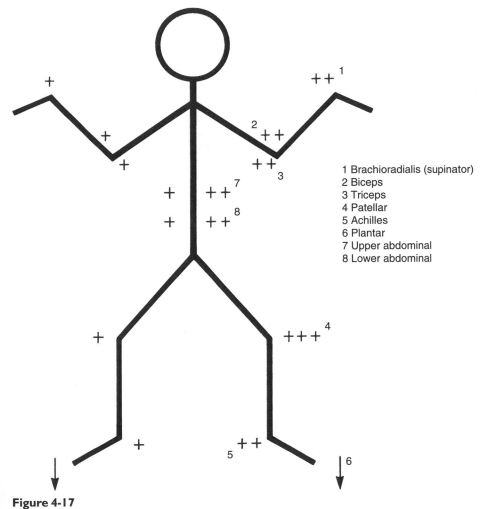

1 Brachioradialis (supinator)
2 Biceps
3 Triceps
4 Patellar
5 Achilles
6 Plantar
7 Upper abdominal
8 Lower abdominal

Figure 4-17
Documentation of Reflexes.
Stick figures are used to document the reflexes. The pluses, indicative of the briskness of the response, are placed close to the position of the reflex. The down-going arrows indicate normal down-going toes.

TABLE 4-12

Reflexes Indicative of Neurologic Pathology

Reflex	Significance
Babinski's (plantar)	Extrapyramidal tract pathology
Snout	Diffuse brain disease
Sucking	Diffuse brain disease
Grasp	Prefrontal lobe lesions
Hoffmann's	Corticospinal tract dysfunction
Oculocephalic	Brainstem pathology
Oculovestibular	Brainstem pathology

oculocephalic reflex, also known as the *doll's eye test*, is elicited by turning the patient's head quickly from side to side. If the brainstem is intact, the eyes move in the opposite direction and maintain the straight-ahead gaze position. If the brainstem is not intact, the eyes move in the direction the head is turned. The oculovestibular reflex also tests brain function. The reflex is elicited by elevating the patient's head about 30 degrees and then instilling cold water in the ear canal. If the brainstem is intact, the normal neurologic response is the development of nystagmus.

TERMINOLOGY

abduction: Movement away from the midline of the body.

abstract reasoning: The ability to think beyond concrete terms

acalcula: The inability to calculate

adduction: Movement toward the midline of the body

affect: The observed emotion

agraphia: The inability to write

anosmia: Complete loss of the sense of smell

anosognosia: The inability to recognize one's own impairment

aphasia: The inability to speak

aphonia: The loss of voice

asterixis: Involuntary movements characterized by nonrhythmic flapping of the extremities

athetosis: Involuntary movements characterized by slow, twisting irregular motions

attention: The ability to focus on one activity

blocking: An abnormal thought process characterized by sudden interruption of speech in midsentence

chorea: Involuntary movement characterized by brief, rapid, irregular, jerky motions

circumstantiality: An abnormal thought process characterized by unnecessary detail that delays reaching the point of the thought

clanging: An abnormal thought process characterized by the use of words on the basis of sound instead of meaning

clonus: Rhythmic oscillation between extension and flexion

coma: An altered state of consciousness characterized by complete loss of consciousness, unresponsiveness to stimuli, and absence of voluntary movement

confabulation: An abnormal thought process characterized by fabrication of facts or events to fill gaps in the memory

confusion: An abnormality of consciousness characterized by mental slowness, inattentiveness, and incoherent thought patterns

decerebrate rigidity: An abnormal body position observed in comatose patients characterized by clenched jaws, extension of the neck and legs, adduction of the arms, pronation of the forearms, and flexion of the wrists and fingers

decorticate rigidity: An abnormal body position observed in comatose patients characterized by flexion of the fingers and wrists and extension and internal rotation of the legs

delirium: An abnormality of consciousness characterized by confusion, agitation, and hallucinations

dementia: Acquired memory impairment

dysarthria: Poorly coordinated, irregular speech

dyscalculia: Difficulty calculating

dysgraphia: Difficulty writing

dyslexia: Difficulty reading

dysphasia: Hesitancy and error in choosing words when speaking

dysphonia: Hoarseness

dyspraxia: Difficulty coordinating body movements

dystaxia: Difficulty with muscle coordination

dystonia: Abnormal slow, twisting, irregular movements

echolalia: An abnormal thought process characterized by repetition of words or phrases spoken by others

eversion: The turning of the toes onto the great toe (foot flexed outward)

extension: The bending of a joint to bring the joint parallel to the long axis

fasciculations: Involuntary movements characterized by fine twitching that rarely moves a joint

flexion: The bending of a joint to bring the parts of the joint into close approximation

flight of ideas: An abnormal thought process characterized by an almost continuous flow of accelerated speech with quick changes of subject

hemianopsia: A visual field defect associated with disorders of the optic chiasm or tract

hemiplegia: Paralysis of one side of the body

incoherence: An abnormal thought process characterized by illogical connections and quick changes of subject

intention tremor: Involuntary movements characterized by tremors that are absent at rest but appear with intentional movement

inversion: The turning of the toes onto the small toes (foot flexed inward)

judgment: The ability to compare and evaluate alternatives

loose associations: Abnormal thought processes characterized by repeated shifting to unrelated subjects

mood: The sustained emotional state

myoclonus: Involuntary movements characterized by sudden, brief, unpredictable jerks

neologism: An abnormal thought process characterized by the use of invented words or the use of words with new meanings

nystagmus: Involuntary oscillation of the eyeball; described as lateral if the eyeball oscillates from side to side, vertical if the eyeball oscillates up and down, and rotatory if the eyeball oscillates in a circle

ophthalmoplegias: Optic movement disorders

paraparesis: A slight degree of lower extremity paralysis

paraplegia: Paralysis of the lower extremities and trunk

perseveration: An abnormal thought process characterized by persistent repetition of words or phrases

postural tremor: Involuntary tremor that occurs when the affected part maintains position

pronation: To place in a downward-facing position.

quadriplegia: Paralysis of the upper and lower extremities

recent memory: Memory of information of a few hours or days

remote memory: Memory of information from the distant past

resting or static tremor: Involuntary movement at rest

scotoma: A visual field defect associated with disorders of the optic nerve

stereognosis: The ability to identify, by touch, small objects placed in the hand

stupor: An abnormal state of consciousness characterized by reduced mental and physical activity and response to stimuli

supination: To place in an upward-facing position

thought content: What a person thinks about

tics: Involuntary movements characterized by brief, repetitive movements at irregular intervals

SELF-ASSESSMENT QUESTIONS

1. Which one of the following abbreviation/interpretation pairs is incorrect?
   a. A&P—auscultation and percussion
   b. NCAT—normocephalic atraumatic
   c. RRR—regular rate and rhythm
   d. CTA—clear to auscultation
   e. MSE—minor system examination

2. The term hyperopia means which of the following?
   a. Nearsightedness
   b. Increased intraocular pressure
   c. Farsightedness
   d. Astigmatism
   e. Abnormal protrusion of the eyeball

3. Which one of the following is not a fundamental physical assessment technique?
   a. Percussion
   b. Inspection
   c. Auscultation
   d. Survey
   e. Palpation

4. Which one of the following apertures is used to assess undilated pupils?
   a. Wide angle
   b. Intermediate
   c. Red free
   d. Slit
   e. Fixation target

5. Nails and nail beds are evaluated for which of the following?
   a. Clubbing
   b. Cyanosis
   c. Trauma
   d. All of the above
   e. None of the above

6. Which of the following best describes the smell of the breath of a patient with severe liver disease?
   a. Fruity
   b. Urinous
   c. Alcoholic
   d. Sweet
   e. Musty

7. On the anterior view, where is the apex of the lung located?
   a. About 3 to 4 cm above the medial end of the clavicles
   b. Between the sixth and eighth ribs
   c. Even with the clavicles
   d. Below the tenth thoracic vertebra
   e. About 3 to 4 cm below the lateral end of the clavicles

8. A patient's muscle strength is noted to be "5+." What does this mean?
   a. No muscle contractility
   b. Barely detectable muscle contractility
   c. Active muscle contractility; able to work against gravity and full resistance
   d. Active muscle contractility; able to work against gravity but not resistance
   e. Active muscle contractility; able to work against gravity and some resistance

9. The normal liver span along the midclavicular line is how long?
   a. 5 cm
   b. 7 cm
   c. 10 cm
   d. 14 cm
   e. 20 cm

10. Interpretation of common proverbs assesses which of the following?
    a. Long-term memory
    b. Abstract thinking
    c. Judgment
    d. Praxis
    e. Affect

Review of Laboratory and Diagnostic Tests

5
CHAPTER

Learning Objectives

- Differentiate between invasive and noninvasive tests.
- State the clinical application of common general diagnostic procedures.
- Identify the clinical application of specific laboratory tests.
- Identify the clinical application of specific diagnostic procedures.
- Assess common laboratory and diagnostic test results.

D ata from laboratory and diagnostic tests and procedures provide important information regarding the response to drug therapy, the ability of patients to metabolize and eliminate specific therapeutic agents, the diagnosis of disease, and the progression and regression of disease.

This chapter reviews the laboratory and diagnostic tests commonly encountered in the patient care environment. The tests are presented using an organ system approach (i.e., cardiovascular, endocrine, gastrointestinal, hematologic, immunologic, neurologic, renal, and respiratory); separate sections for the assessment of infectious diseases and nutritional status are included. More detailed information about these and other laboratory and diagnostic tests is available in laboratory and medicine textbooks and the current literature.

BACKGROUND

Laboratory and diagnostic tests are classified as either *invasive* or *noninvasive* tests. *Invasive* tests are those that require penetration of the skin or insertion of instruments or devices into a body orifice. The degree of risk with invasive tests varies from relatively minor risks such as the pain, bleeding, and bruising associated with venipuncture to the risk of death associated with more invasive procedures such as coronary angiography. Examples of invasive tests include collection of blood (venipuncture), insertion of a central venous catheter, and collection of cerebrospinal fluid. *Noninvasive* tests do not penetrate the skin or involve insertion of instruments into body orifices and pose little risk to the patient. Examples of noninvasive tests include the chest radiograph, analysis of spontaneously voided urine, and stool occult blood analysis.

The selection of specific tests and procedures depends on the patient's underlying condition, the need for the information, and the degree of risk. For example, venipuncture may be considered too invasive for patients with chronic, stable disease, but it may be an essential risk when initiating drug treatment in a patient with unstable disease.

Reference ranges are listed in Tables 5-1 through 5-7.[1-3] Individual laboratory test results are interpreted using laboratory-specific reference ranges. Reference ranges may differ among different laboratories depending on the population and laboratory methodology used to establish the range. Statistically derived reference ranges encompass the tested mean ±2 standard deviations. This means that 1 in 20 normal test results fall outside the reference range.

Factors to consider when interpreting individual test results include patient age, gender, timing of the test result in relationship to drug administration, concomitant drug therapy, concurrent diseases, organ function (e.g., renal function, liver function, cardiac function), test sensitivity (the proportion of true-positive results), test specificity (the proportion of true-negative results), timing of the test in relation to drug dosing or known circadian rhythms, genetics (e.g., glucose-6-phosphate deficiency), and fluid status (e.g., euvolemia, dehydration, fluid overload). Refer to laboratory textbooks or the published literature for detailed discussions of these factors.

GENERAL ORGAN SYSTEM MONITORING

A variety of tests and procedures are used to diagnosis and monitor conditions that affect various organ systems. The applications and uses of these tests and procedures continue to expand with experience and the integration of new technology.

LABORATORY TESTS AND DIAGNOSTIC PROCEDURES

Angiography.   Angiography is a radiographic test used to evaluate blood vessels and the circulation. Radiopaque material is injected through a catheter, and images are recorded using standard radiographic techniques.

Biopsy.   A biopsy involves the removal and evaluation of tissue.

Computed Tomography.   Computed tomography (CT; CAT scan) uses a computerized x-ray system to produce detailed sectional x-ray images. The system is very sensitive to differences in tissue density and produces detailed, two-dimensional planar images; contrast agents increase attenuation. The spiral or helical CT takes pictures continuously, decreasing the time needed to obtain images.

Doppler Echography.   Doppler echography uses ultrasound technology to measure shifts in frequency from moving images. For example, Doppler echography is used to evaluate blood flow velocity and turbulence in the heart (Doppler echocardiography) and peripheral circulation.

Endoscopy.   Endoscopy is used to examine the interior of a hollow viscus (e.g., digestive, respiratory, and urogenital organs and the endocrine system) or canal (e.g., bile ducts, pancreas). The endoscope, a flexible or inflexible tube with a camera and light source, is inserted into a body orifice (Figure 5-1). Still and/or video images are recorded and tissues obtained for biopsy or other laboratory diagnostic tests.

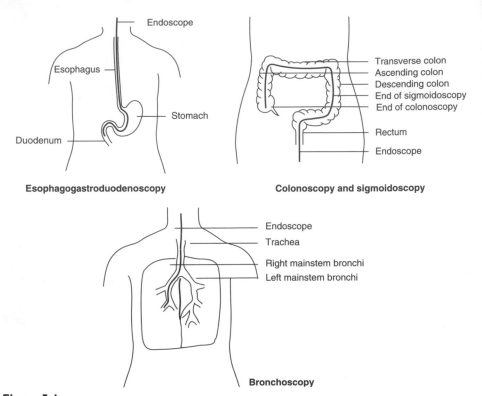

Figure 5-1
Endoscopy.
Endoscopy is performed to evaluate the inside of hollow body organs or canals.

Examples of common endoscopic procedures include colonoscopy (views the inside of the entire colon from rectum to end of the small intestine), sigmoidoscopy (views the inside of the large intestine from the rectum through the sigmoid colon), cholangiopancreatography (views the inside of the bile ducts and pancreas), esophagogastroduodenoscopy (views the inside of the esophagus, stomach, and duodenum), and bronchoscopy (views the inside of the tracheobronchial tree).

Fluoroscopy.   Fluoroscopy uses a fluoroscope, a device that makes the shadows of x-ray films visible, to provide real-time visualization of procedures. Fluoroscopy exposes a patient to more radiation than routine radiography but often is used to guide needle biopsy procedures and nasogastric tube advancement.

Magnetic Resonance Imaging.   Magnetic resonance imaging (MRI) uses an externally applied magnetic field to align the axis of nuclear spin of cellular nuclei. The patient is surrounded by the magnetic field (Figure 5-2). Brief radiofrequency pulses are applied to displace the alignment. The energy emitted when the displacement ends is detected, resulting in finely detailed planar and three-dimensional images; contrast agents increase the attenuation.

Paracentesis.   Paracentesis is the removal and analysis of fluid from a body cavity.

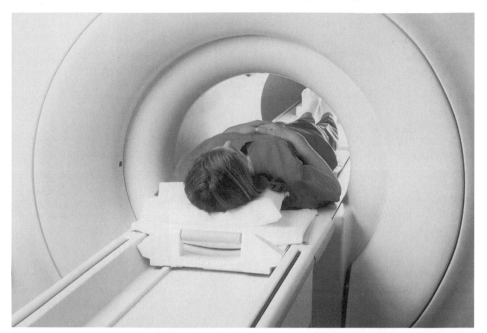

Figure 5-2
Magnetic Resonance Imaging.
Magnetic resonance imaging (MRI) uses an externally applied magnetic field to obtain detailed images of anatomic structures. (Courtesy General Electric Medical Systems.)

Plethysmography.   Plethysmography measures changes in the size of vessels and hollow organs by measuring displacement of air or fluid from a containment system. Body plethysmography is used to assess pulmonary function.

Positron Emission Tomography.   Positron emission tomography (PET) imaging uses positron-emitting radionuclides to visualize organs and tissues of the body. The radionuclides decay, producing positrons that collide with electrons. A special camera detects photons, released when the positrons and electrons collide. PET imaging provides quantitative information regarding the structure and function of organs and tissues.

Radionuclide Studies.   Radionuclide studies involve the administration of oral, parenteral, or inhaled radioactive chemicals or pharmaceuticals. X-ray images, usually serial, record the collection and dispersion of the radioactive material. The ventilation/perfusion scan of the lungs is an example of a radionuclide study.

Single-Photon Emission Computed Tomography.   Single-photon emission computed tomography (SPECT) is similar to PET but involves the administration of radionuclides that emit gamma rays. SPECT is less expensive than PET but provides more limited image resolution.

Standard Radiography (Plain Films, X-Ray Films).   Standard radiography produces images on photographic plates by passing roentgen rays through the body

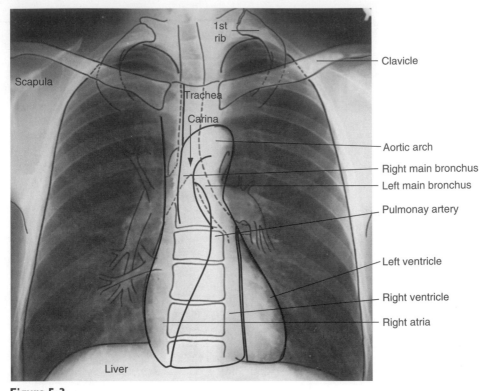

Figure 5-3
Chest Radiography.
Chest radiography is used to assess chest structures.

(Figure 5-3). These films are sometimes difficult to interpret because the three dimensionality is lost on the planar images.

Ultrasonography (Echography).   Ultrasonography uses ultrasound (high-frequency sound waves imperceptible to the human ear) to create images of organs and vessels. For example, ultrasonography is used to visualize the fetus in utero.

CARDIOVASCULAR SYSTEM

A variety of noninvasive and invasive laboratory and diagnostic tests are used to evaluate and monitor the cardiovascular system. Cardiovascular reference ranges are listed in Table 5-1.

LABORATORY TESTS
Cardiac Enzymes.   The pattern and time course of the appearance of enzymes in the blood after cardiac muscle cell damage are used to diagnose myocardial infarction.[4]
   Creatine Kinase.   Creatine kinase (CK; creatine phosphokinase) is found in skeletal muscle; cardiac muscle; and the brain, bladder, stomach, and colon. Isoenzyme fractions identify the type of tissue damaged. CK-BB (CK1) is found in

TABLE 5-1

Adult Cardiovascular Laboratory Reference Values (Based on Serum Tests)

Index	Reference Range
Creatine kinase	
Female	40-150 U/L
Male	60-400 U/L
CK-MB	0-7.5 ng/ml
C-reactive protein	<8 µg/ml
Lactic dehydrogenase	110-210 U/L
Lactic dehydrogenase isoenzymes	
LDH_1	17%-27%
LDH_2	28%-38%
LDH_3	18%-28%
LDH_4	5%-15%
LDH_5	5%-15%
Lipids	
Cholesterol	<200 mg/dl
Triglycerides (fasting)	40-150 mg/dl
Troponins	
Troponin I	<0.35 ng/ml
Troponin T	<0.2 µg/L

From Jordan CD et al: N Engl J Med 327:718-724, 1992; Sacher RA, McPherson RA: *Widmann's clinical interpretation of laboratory tests*, ed 11, Philadelphia, 2000, FA Davis; and Tilkian SM, Conover MB, Tilkian AG: *Clinical nursing implications of laboratory tests*, ed 5, St Louis, 1996, Mosby.

the brain, bladder, stomach, and colon; CK-MB (CK2) is found in cardiac tissue; and CK-MM (CK3) is found in skeletal muscle. CK-MB is detected in the blood within 3 to 5 hours after a myocardial infarction; levels peak in about 10 to 20 hours and normalize within about 3 days.

Lactic Dehydrogenase. Lactic dehydrogenase (LDH) is found in a variety of body tissues. Isoenzyme fractions are used to identify the type of tissue damage. LDH_1 and LDH_2 are found in the heart, brain, and erythrocytes. LDH_3 is found in the brain and kidneys. LDH_4 is found in the liver, skeletal muscle, and kidneys. LDH_5 is found in the liver, skeletal muscle, and ileum. LDH_2 normally accounts for the highest percentage of total serum LDH. After a myocardial infarction the rise in LDH_1 concentration exceeds the rise in LDH_2 concentration (the LDH_1-to-LDH_2 ratio is >1; a "flipped" ratio). LDH increases within about 12 hours after a myocardial infarction, peaks between 24 and 48 hours, and normalizes by about day 10.

Cholesterol. Cholesterol is separated into lipoproteins by protein electrophoresis. Low-density lipoprotein (LDL) is strongly correlated with coronary artery disease. High-density lipoprotein (HDL) is inversely correlated with coronary artery disease.

C-Reactive Protein. C-reactive protein is a biologic marker of systemic inflammation. Preliminary studies have linked an increased C-reactive protein concentration with an increased risk of myocardial infarction, stroke, and peripheral arterial disease.

Myoglobin.   Myoglobin is a small protein found in cardiac and skeletal muscle. The presence of myoglobin in the urine or plasma is a relatively sensitive indicator of cellular damage.

Triglycerides.   Triglycerides are found in very-low-density lipoproteins (VLDLs) and chylomicrons.

Troponins.   Troponins are a complex of proteins (troponin I, C, and T) that mediate the actin and myosin interaction in muscle. Troponins I and T are specific to cardiac muscle and are used to identify cardiac muscle injury. Troponin I and T concentrations increase within a few hours of cardiac muscle injury and remain elevated for 5 to 7 days.

DIAGNOSTIC TESTS AND PROCEDURES

Cardiac Catheterization.   Cardiac catheterization is used to evaluate cardiac function.[5] A catheter is passed into the right or left side of the heart. Transducers on the tip of the catheter record pressures in the vessels and chambers of the heart. Ports in the catheter provide access for blood samples for the determination of oxygen content and cardiac output.[6] Right-sided catheterization is used to measure right atrial pressures, right ventricular pressures, pulmonary artery pressures, and pulmonary artery occlusion pressure. Left-sided catheterization is used to measure left ventricular pressures.

Central Line Placement with Hemodynamic Monitoring.   A catheter is placed into the central venous system and advanced into the right side of the heart (Figure 5-4). The right atrial, right ventricular, pulmonary artery, and pulmonary artery occlusion (formerly known as the *pulmonary capillary wedge*) pressures are measured, and cardiac output is calculated. These parameters are used to monitor the hemodynamic status of the patient and to calculate the pulmonary and peripheral vascular resistances.

Chest Radiography.   Chest x-ray films are used to diagnose cardiac disease and monitor the patient's response to drug and nondrug therapy (see Figure 5-3). The chest radiograph is used to determine the size and shape of the atria and ventricles, to calculate the cardiothoracic ratio, and to detect abnormalities in the lung fields and pleural spaces.

Coronary Angiography.   In coronary angiography the cardiac vessels are visualized by injecting the vessel with a contrast agent.

Digital Subtraction Angiography.   In digital subtraction angiography (DSA), background images are obtained before the contrast agent is injected. The background images are then "subtracted" from the images obtained after the injection of the contrast agent. This technique improves image resolution.

Echocardiography.   Echocardiography is used to evaluate the size, shape, and motion of the valves, septum, and walls and changes in chamber size during the cardiac cycle.[7] The beam is applied to the heart through the chest (transthoracic approach) or esophagus (transesophageal approach).
   Contrast Echocardiography.   Visualization of the right-sided chambers of the heart is enhanced by the injection of contrast agents.

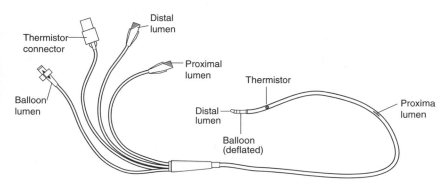

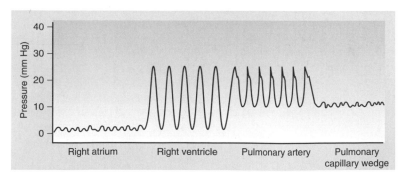

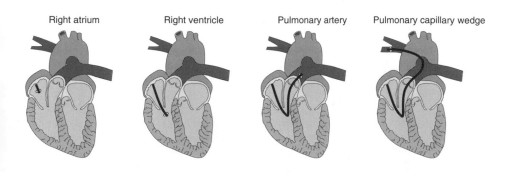

Figure 5-4
Swan-Ganz Catheterization.
Pulmonary artery catheter, catheter positions in the heart, and typical pressure waveforms.

Doppler Echocardiography. Doppler and echocardiography techniques are combined to evaluate cardiac blood flow patterns.

Exercise Echocardiography. Exercise echocardiography compares echocardiograms obtained before and during exercise.

M-Mode Echocardiography.   M-mode echocardiography records the motion of the heart over time. It is used to evaluate the structures of the heart throughout the cardiac cycle.

Two-Dimensional Echocardiography.   Two-dimensional echocardiography records a two-dimensional image of the heart. The spatial anatomic relationships can be determined by changing the angle of the beam.

Electrocardiography.   Electrocardiography records cardiac electrical activity.

Electrocardiogram.   The electrocardiogram (ECG) records the electrical activity of the heart (Figure 5-5).[8] The ECG is used to diagnose cardiac disease, monitor the patient's response to drug therapy, and monitor for adverse drug effects. Twelve separate leads, six extremity (limb) leads (aVR [augmented voltage right arm], aVL [augmented voltage left arm], aVF [augmented voltage left foot], I, II, III) and six chest (precordial) leads (V1, V2, V3, V4, V5, V6) create a three-dimensional view of cardiac electrical activity.

Electrocardiogram with Stress (Stress Test).   The ECG is recorded during a standardized exercise protocol with gradually increasing levels of exercise[9,10] or with the

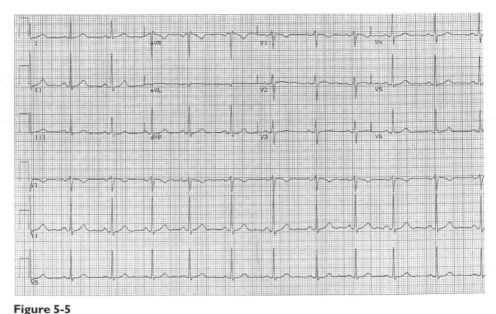

26–DEC–92 09:27   ROUT RETRII

25mm/s	Med: unknown
10mm/mV	04–MAR–30 Ht : Wt:
100Hz	Sex: F Race: Blk
Pgm 004C	Loc: 1 Room : ER 3
12SL v78	Option: 1

NORMAL SINUS RHYTHM—Computer interprotation
NORMAL ECG

Vent. Rate   66 BPM
PR interval   172   ms
QRS duration   96   ms
QT/QTc   416/429   ms
P-R-T axes   78 61   53

Matrix of information.
Computer measurement
of intervals and durations

Figure 5-5
12-Lead Electrocardiogram.
Normal 12-lead electrocardiogram. (From Phalen T: *The 12-lead ECG in acute myocardial infarction*, St Louis, 1996, Mosby.)

patient at rest after the administration of dobutamine or dipyridamole; either intervention increases myocardial oxygen consumption and blood flow. A motorized treadmill or cycle ergometer is used for the exercise stress test. Blood pressure, heart rate, oxygen consumption, oxygen saturation, and arterial blood gas data are commonly collected to provide a thorough assessment of how the cardiovascular system functions under stress conditions.

Holter Monitoring (Ambulatory Electrocardiography). The Holter monitor is a portable recorder used to record the ECG continuously throughout usual patient activity.

Thallium Stress Test. The thallium stress test combines the parenteral administration of thallium-201, a radionuclide taken up by healthy myocardial tissue, and the stress test (either exercise or pharmacologic). A gamma camera is used to record serial images of the myocardium.

Intracardiac Electrophysiologic Studies. Intracardiac electrophysiologic studies (EPSs) are tests in which special catheters with electrodes are used to stimulate the cardiac tissue to assess the nature and origin of cardiac arrhythmias and the response to antiarrhythmic drug therapy.

Lymphoscintigraphy. Lymphoscintigraphy evaluates the patency and anatomy of peripheral lymph vessels by depositing a radioactive agent in the tissue drained by the lymph system being evaluated.[11,12] The test is used to assess lymphedema and tumor involvement of regional lymph nodes inaccessible to other imaging procedures.

Multiple Gated Acquisition Scan. The multiple gated acquisition (MUGA) scan, also known as *radionuclide angiocardiography,* evaluates ventricular function, cardiac wall motion, ejection fraction, and cardiac output after the injection of radionuclide-labeled (technetium-99m) albumin or red blood cells (RBCs).[13]

Technetium-99m Pyrophosphate Uptake. Infarcted myocardial tissue has an increased uptake of technetium-99m compared with healthy tissue. The isotope is injected parenterally, and serial images of the heart are obtained to evaluate the location and extent of the myocardial infarction.

ENDOCRINE SYSTEM

The endocrine system consists of the pituitary, hypothalamus, adrenal gland, thyroid gland, parathyroid glands, and pancreas. The endocrine system is assessed by measuring the levels of the hormones produced by the different components of the system.[14,15] Therapeutic response to replacement or suppressive drug therapy also is assessed by measuring the levels of these hormones. A variety of specific tests are used to assess each component of the endocrine system. Endocrine reference ranges are listed in Table 5-2.

LABORATORY TESTS
Adrenal Tests

Adrenal Medulla. The adrenal medulla secretes catecholamines. The 24-hour urinary excretion of epinephrine, norepinephrine, and vanillylmandelic acid (VMA) is used to assess the function of the adrenal medulla.

Adrenal Cortex. The adrenal cortex secretes mineralocorticoids, glucocorticoids, and androgens. Tests used to assess the function of the adrenal cortex include plasma

TABLE 5-2

Adult Endocrine Laboratory Reference Values

Index	Source	Reference Range
Thyroid		
Free thyroxine index		4.6-11.2
Thyroid-stimulating hormone	S	0.5-5 µU/ml
Total triiodothyronine (T_3)	S	75-195 ng/dl
Total thyroxine (T_4)	S	4-12 µg/dl
Pituitary		
Adrenocorticotropic hormone (ACTH)	P	6-76 pg/ml
Growth hormone (fasting)	P	2-6 ng/ml
Prolactin		
Female	S	0-15 ng/ml
Male	S	0-10 ng/ml
Adrenal Cortex		
Aldosterone (recumbent, normal salt diet)	S, P	<16 ng/dl
Cortisol (8 AM fasting)	P	0-10 µg/dl
Renin (supine) (6 hr, recumbent, normal salt diet)	P	0.5-1.6 ng/ml/hr
Adrenal Medulla and Catechol Secretions		
Epinephrine	U	1.7-22.4 µg/day
Norepinephrine	U	12.1-85.5 µg/day
Vanillylmandelic acid (VMA)	U	1.4-6.5 mg/day
Gonadal Hormones		
Estradiol		
Female		
Premenopausal	S, P	23-361 pg/ml
Postmenopausal	S, P	<30 pg/ml
Male	S, P	<50 pg/ml
Testosterone		
Female	P	20-90 ng/dl
Male	P	300-1100 ng/dl
Pancreatic		
Amylase	S	53-123 U/L
Glucose (fasting)	P	70-110 mg/dl
Insulin (fasting)	S	0-29 µU/ml
Lipase	S	4-24 U/dl
Parathyroid		
Calcium	S	8.5-10.5 mg/dl
Parathyroid hormone	P	10-60 pg/ml
Phosphorus	S	2.6-4.5 mg/dl

From Jordan CD et al: N Engl J Med 327:718-724, 1992; Sacher RA, McPherson RA: *Widmann's clinical interpretation of laboratory tests*, ed 11, Philadelphia, 2000, FA Davis; and Tilkian SM, Conover MB, Tilkian AG: *Clinical nursing implications of laboratory tests*, ed 5, St Louis, 1996, Mosby.
P, Plasma; S, serum; U, urine.

and urine aldosterone; plasma renin activity; serum testosterone; serum estradiol; plasma cortisol (morning and evening); plasma adrenocorticotropic hormone (ACTH) (morning); and urinary excretion rates of the 17-hydroxycorticosteroids, 17-ketogenic steroids, and 17-ketosteroids.

Dexamethasone Suppression Test. Dexamethasone suppresses ACTH secretion. A baseline 8 AM plasma cortisol level is obtained and then 1 mg of dexamethasone is administered orally at 11 PM. Normally, cortisol production is suppressed, and the 8 AM plasma cortisol level obtained the next day is low.

Human Chorionic Gonadotropin.   Human chorionic gonadotropin (hCG) is produced by the placenta. It is detected in the urine as early as 10 days after a missed menstrual cycle and peaks at about 10 weeks.

Insulin Tolerance Test.   Insulin (0.05 to 0.1 U/kg) is administered intravenously. Serial blood samples are obtained for 90 minutes. ACTH is released when the blood glucose falls to less than 40 mg/dl.

Metyrapone Test.   Metyrapone inhibits the final step in cortisol synthesis. For this test, 500 to 750 mg of metyrapone is administered orally every 4 hours for 24 hours and plasma samples are collected. A normal response is a decrease in plasma cortisol and an elevation in urine and plasma 11-deoxycortisol (compound S).

Pancreatic Tests

Amylase.   Amylase is secreted by the pancreas, bowel, parotids, and gynecologic system. Although not specific for pancreatitis, serum amylase is easier to measure than is lipase and is used as a common screening and monitoring parameter for acute pancreatitis. However, in chronic pancreatitis the pancreas may be "burned out" and unable to secrete amylase.

C Peptide.   C peptide is an inactive peptide chain released from beta cells in equimolar amounts with insulin and found in the serum in about a 5:1 to 15:1 ratio with insulin. C peptide is sometimes used to assess pancreatic function.

Glucose.   Serum glucose concentrations are used to assess pancreatic function and the response to insulin replacement therapy.

Fasting Serum Glucose.   The serum sample is obtained after 10 to 14 hours of fasting. The fasting serum glucose is usually obtained before breakfast after an overnight fast.

Glucose Tolerance Test.   The glucose tolerance test (GTT) is used to diagnose diabetes mellitus and gestational diabetes. Patients fast for 10 to 16 hours before the test and are then given approximately 75 g of glucose. Serial blood samples are obtained, and the serum glucose concentration is determined. Normally, the serum blood glucose is less than 200 mg/dl at 30, 60, and 90 minutes and less than 140 mg/dl at 2 hours.

Random Serum Glucose.   The random serum glucose sample can be obtained at any time without fasting.

Glycosylated Hemoglobin.   Glycosylated hemoglobin is formed when hemoglobin is irreversibly glycosylated after exposure to high glucose levels. Glycosylated hemoglobin assesses long-term control of insulin therapy and differentiates factitious hyperglycemia from diabetes.

Insulin.   Fasting serum insulin is sometimes obtained during the assessment of pancreatic function.

Lipase. Lipase is a specific marker for acute pancreatic disease. Increases in serum lipase parallel increases in serum amylase. However, in chronic pancreatitis the pancreas may be "burned out" and unable to secrete lipase.

Parathyroid Tests. The parathyroid gland secretes parathyroid hormone (PTH). High serum calcium levels suppress PTH secretion. Parathyroid gland function is tested by measuring the serum concentrations of PTH, calcium, and phosphorus. The serum concentration of PTH is useful in differentiating between hypercalcemia resulting from hyperparathyroidism and hypercalcemia resulting from other causes.

Pituitary Tests

Anterior Pituitary. The anterior pituitary hormones include growth hormone, prolactin, thyroid-stimulating hormone (TSH), follicle-stimulating hormone, luteinizing hormone, and ACTH. Pituitary function is assessed by measuring the concentrations of the hormones at baseline and after stimulation or suppression tests.

Adrenocorticotropic Hormone Stimulation Test. ACTH stimulates adrenal cortisol production. A baseline plasma cortisol level is obtained and then 250 µg of cosyntropin is injected intravenously. Normally, plasma cortisol levels peak in 30 to 60 minutes.

Posterior Pituitary. The posterior pituitary hormones include antidiuretic hormone and oxytocin. Tests used to evaluate posterior pituitary function include concentration testing and water loading. Concentration testing involves overnight water deprivation and evaluation of urine and serum osmolality. Water loading involves the administration of 1000 ml of water and then evaluation of urine and serum osmolality.

Thyroid Tests. Thyroid function tests are used to establish the level of thyroid function (e.g., hyperthyroid, hypothyroid, euthyroid) and the response to suppressant or replacement therapy. Thyroid function is assessed by evaluating the serum concentrations of the free hormones thyroxine (T_4) and triiodothyronine (T_3) and by a number of indirect methods.

Free Thyroxine Index. The free thyroxine index (FT_4I) is the product of the measured T_4 and the triiodothyronine uptake (T_3U). It takes into account the absolute hormone level and the binding capacity of thyroid-binding globulin. The FT_4I is decreased in hypothyroidism and increased in hyperthyroidism.

Thyroid-Stimulating Hormone (Thyrotropin). Serum TSH, or thyrotropin, levels are used to differentiate between thyroid hypothyroidism and pituitary hypothyroidism. The TSH level is elevated in thyroidal hypothyroidism and markedly decreased in pituitary hypothyroidism.

Thyroid Uptake of Radioiodine. Radioactive iodine (^{123}I or ^{131}I) is administered orally, and the radioactivity over the thyroid gland is counted at various intervals. The normal radioactive iodine uptake (RAIU) is about 10% to 35%.

Thyrotropin-Releasing Hormone. Thyrotropin-releasing hormone (TRH) stimulates the pituitary to release TSH. Injection of synthetic TRH normally causes an increase in TSH in about 30 minutes.

Triiodothyronine Uptake. The triiodothyronine uptake (T_3U) test is an in vitro test that indirectly estimates the amount of thyroid-binding globulin in the serum.

GASTROINTESTINAL SYSTEM

A variety of noninvasive and invasive laboratory and diagnostic tests are used to evaluate and monitor the gastrointestinal system. Gastrointestinal reference ranges are listed in Table 5-3.

LABORATORY TESTS

Biliary System.   Bilirubin is useful in the diagnosis and monitoring of liver disease and hemolytic anemia and in the assessment of the severity of jaundice. A patient is generally visibly jaundiced if the bilirubin level is greater than 2 mg/dl.

   Alkaline Phosphatase.   Alkaline phosphatase is elevated in biliary cirrhosis, cirrhosis, and intrahepatic bile duct disease.

   Direct Bilirubin.   Direct bilirubin is water-soluble conjugated posthepatic bilirubin. It is increased with biliary disease (e.g., extrahepatic bile duct obstruction, physical

---

TABLE 5-3

Adult Gastrointestinal Laboratory Reference Values

Index	Source	Reference Range
Alanine aminotransferase (ALT)		
Female	S	7-30 U/L
Male	S	10-55 U/L
Alkaline phosphatase		
Female	S	30-100 U/L
Male	S	45-115 U/L
Ammonia	P	12-55 µmol/L
Aspartate aminotransferase (AST)		
Female	S	9-25 U/L
Male	S	10-40 U/L
Bilirubin		
Direct	S	Up to 0.4 mg/dl
Total	S	Up to 1 mg/dl
Gamma glutamyl transpeptidase (GGT)	S	1-60 U/L
Lactic dehydrogenase (LDH)	S	110-210 U/L
Partial thromboplastin time, activated (aPTT)	P	24-37 sec
Protein		
Albumin	S	3.1-4.3 g/dl
Globulin	S	2.6-4.1 g/dl
Total	S	6-8 g/dl (60-80 g/L)
Prothrombin time (PT)	P	8.8-11.6 sec
Stool fat	Stool	1-7 g/day

From Jordan CD et al: N Engl J Med 327:718-724, 1992; Sacher RA, McPherson RA: *Widmann's clinical interpretation of laboratory tests*, ed 11, Philadelphia, 2000, FA Davis; and Tilkian SM, Conover MB, Tilkian AG: *Clinical nursing implications of laboratory tests*, ed 5, St Louis, 1996, Mosby.
P, Plasma; S, serum.

impairment of bile flow, impaired bile transport) and some liver disease (e.g., hepatitis, cirrhosis, hepatic neoplasm).

Delta Bilirubin.   Delta bilirubin is albumin-bound conjugated bilirubin. A calculated value [delta bilirubin = total bilirubin − (unconjugated bilirubin + conjugated bilirubin)], delta bilirubin is metabolically inactive and cleared slowly from the body. Delta bilirubin is increased with biliary obstruction and some liver disease.

Indirect Bilirubin.   Indirect bilirubin is unconjugated bilirubin. It is increased with hemolytic anemia (rapid, severe hemolysis) and some liver disease.

Total Bilirubin.   Total bilirubin is the sum of all three forms of bilirubin (direct bilirubin, indirect bilirubin, and delta bilirubin). Total bilirubin is increased with hepatic and hemolytic disease.

Hepatic Synthetic Function.   Many drugs are hepatically metabolized. One way of assessing the liver's ability to metabolize these agents is to assess the synthetic function of the liver by evaluating the quantity of specific products produced or processed by the liver.[16] These include ammonia, albumin, and the vitamin K–dependent clotting factors.

Ammonia.   The liver synthesizes urea from ammonia. Serum ammonia is increased if the liver is damaged or if blood flow is compromised. Although the serum ammonia is not used as a routine screening test, it is sometimes used to confirm a diagnosis of hepatic encephalopathy.

Protein Production.   The liver manufactures many different proteins. The serum albumin and the vitamin K–dependent clotting factors are commonly used to assess hepatic synthetic function.

Albumin.   Although circulating albumin takes several weeks to clear from the body, a rapidly declining serum protein level indicates greatly impaired hepatic function. Long-standing liver disease is associated with very low serum protein concentrations.

Vitamin K–Dependent Clotting Factors (Factors II, VII, IX, and X).   Lack of production of the vitamin K–dependent clotting factors prolongs the prothrombin time (PT) and partial thromboplastin time (PTT). The PT is prolonged earlier than the PTT and often is used as an early indicator of impaired hepatic synthetic function. Both the PT and PTT are prolonged in long-standing severe hepatic dysfunction.

Hepatocellular Enzymes.   Hepatocytes contain numerous enzymes that leak into the serum when liver cells die or are damaged.[17]

Elevations occur in the presence of marked changes in hepatic circulation (e.g., cardiovascular shock) and diseases associated with hepatocellular damage (hepatitis, cirrhosis, inflammatory diseases, and infiltrative hepatic diseases). However, serum enzymes may not be markedly elevated in severe, chronic, end-stage liver disease (i.e., the liver is "burned out"). Very high elevations (more than 20 times normal) are associated with viral or toxic hepatitis. Moderately high elevations (3 to 10 times normal) are associated with infectious mononucleosis, chronic active hepatitis, extrahepatic bile duct obstruction, and intrahepatic cholestasis. Modest elevations (one to three times normal) are associated with pancreatitis, alcoholic fatty liver, biliary cirrhosis, and neoplastic infiltration.

Alanine Aminotransferase.   Alanine aminotransferase (ALT) is found in high concentrations in hepatocytes and is considered a specific marker of hepatocellular damage.

Aspartate Aminotransferase.   Aspartate aminotransferase (AST) is found in hepatocytes, myocardial muscles, skeletal muscle, the brain, and the kidneys. It is used as a nonspecific marker of hepatocellular damage.

Gamma Glutamyl Transpeptidase.   Gamma glutamyl transpeptidase (GGT) is found in hepatobiliary, pancreatic, and kidney cells. It is elevated in most hepatocellular and hepatobiliary diseases, although elevations correlate better with obstructive disease than with pure hepatocellular damage. An elevated GGT level is an early indicator of alcoholic liver disease.

Lactic Dehydrogenase.   LDH is found in the heart, brain, erythrocytes, kidneys, liver, skeletal muscle, and ileum. Elevations occur during shock syndrome (marked changes in circulation) and diseases associated with hepatocellular damage (hepatitis, cirrhosis, inflammatory disease, and infiltrative diseases).

Stool.   The stool is evaluated for color; consistency; and the presence of obvious or occult blood, fat, ova and parasites, microorganisms, and white blood cells (WBCs). The color of the stool provides important diagnostic and monitoring information. Black stools may indicate upper gastrointestinal tract bleeding; however, iron therapy may produce a similar color. Gray stools are generally associated with steatorrhea; light gray stools may indicate bile duct obstruction. Watery stools are indicative of rapid gastrointestinal transit and malabsorption syndromes. Hard stools may indicate dehydration. The presence of obvious blood in the stool indicates colonic bleeding. Occult blood, present with both upper and lower gastrointestinal tract bleeding, may be identified for several weeks after gastrointestinal bleeding. Stool fat is increased in diseases associated with altered bacterial flora, increased gastrointestinal motility, decreased enzyme and bile acid content, and loss of absorptive surfaces. WBCs are associated with a variety of infectious processes and inflammatory bowel disease.

Miscellaneous

Alpha-Fetoprotein.   Alpha-fetoprotein is the major protein produced by the fetus in the first 10 weeks of life. It also is produced by rapidly multiplying hepatocytes and is used as a marker of hepatocellular carcinoma.

Carcinoembryonic Antigen.   The carcinoembryonic antigen (CEA) is a tumor marker found in the blood. It is associated with rapid multiplication of digestive system epithelial cells and is used to monitor tumor recurrence.

DIAGNOSTIC TESTS AND PROCEDURES

Abdominal Radiography.   The abdominal x-ray film, including the kidneys, ureter, and bladder (KUB), is taken with the patient lying supine on the back.

Barium Studies.   The patient swallows contrast material, such as barium sulfate, and x-ray films are taken to visualize the esophagus, stomach, and small intestine. Barium enemas are used to visualize the large intestine. The double-contrast barium enema technique uses the combination of barium and air to visualize the large intestine and is considered a more precise procedure.

Capsule Endoscopy.   Capsule endoscopy is a relatively new method used to visualize the gastrointestinal tract. The patient swallows a disposable capsule about the size of a large vitamin tablet that contains a miniature video camera, a light source, a miniature transmitter, an antenna, and a battery. Images are transmitted to an external receiver in a belt worn around the patient's waist. Peristalsis moves the capsule through the gastrointestinal system; the capsule is excreted rectally.

Cholecystosonography.   Sonography is used to detect gallstones and evaluate the gallbladder, biliary system, and adjacent organs. Sonography has nearly replaced cholecystography.

Cholecystography.   Cholecystography is used to evaluate gallbladder function and anatomy. Orally administered iopanoic acid concentrates in the gallbladder, opacifying it.[18]

Colonoscopy.   A flexible fiberoptic tube is inserted rectally to visualize the lining of the large intestine from the rectum through the colon to the lower end of the small intestine.

D-Xylose Test.   The D-xylose test is used to screen for carbohydrate malabsorption.[19] For this test a dose of 25 g of D-xylose is administered with water and the urine is collected for a 5-hour period. Normally, more than 3 g of D-xylose is excreted in the urine during this period; lower amounts indicate impaired carbohydrate absorption.

Endoscopic Retrograde Cholangiopancreatography.   Endoscopic retrograde cholangiopancreatography (ERCP) combines endoscopy and x-ray films to visualize the biliary system and pancreas. The endoscope is inserted in the esophagus and advanced to where the bile ducts and pancreas open in the duodenum; contrast dye is injected into the ducts. X-ray films are taken to visualize the ducts.

Endoscopy.   A flexible fiberoptic tube is inserted orally to visualize the lining of the upper and lower gastrointestinal system.

Esophagogastroduodenoscopy.   An endoscope is inserted into the esophagus to visualize the inside of the esophagus, stomach, and duodenum.

Intragastric pH.   The pH of gastric secretions is sometimes measured to monitor the effectiveness of antacid or H_2-receptor antagonist drug therapy.

Manometry.   Manometry is used to evaluate esophageal contractions and esophageal sphincter pressures.[20] Pressures are measured by pressure transducers on a tube inserted orally.

Percutaneous Transhepatic Cholangiogram.   Contrast media is injected directly into the biliary radicle within the liver, and fluoroscopy is used to visualize the intrahepatic and extrahepatic bile ducts.

pH Stimulation Tests.   Tests involving pH stimulation are used to determine the response of gastric acid secretion to a chemical stimulus; they are sometimes used to diagnose hyposecretory and hypersecretory gastric acid disorders. Gastric secretions are collected from the stomach by aspiration through a nasogastric tube. Secretions are collected at baseline and after stimulation with betazole or pentagastrin.

Schilling Test.   The Schilling test is used to evaluate the absorption of vitamin B_{12} (cyanocobalamin). In the first part of the test, 1000 µg of regular B_{12} is administered parenterally to saturate the systemic vitamin B_{12} storage sites. A 0.5- to 1-µg dose of ^{57}Co-labeled vitamin B_{12} is then administered orally, and urine is collected.

Normally, more than 7% of the radiolabeled vitamin B_{12} is excreted in the urine in a 24-hour period. If indicated, the test may be repeated with the administration of 60 μg of oral intrinsic factor. If the malabsorption of vitamin B_{12} is caused by a deficiency of intrinsic factor, the amount of radiolabeled B_{12} excreted in the urine rises to normal levels.

Sigmoidoscopy.   An endoscope is used to evaluate the gastrointestinal tract from the anus to about 60 cm of the terminal colon. The rigid sigmoidoscope is used to screen for rectosigmoid cancer, to obtain large mucosal biopsies, and to evaluate patients with inflammatory disease of the rectum or distal sigmoid colon. The flexible sigmoidoscope is longer and more useful in the assessment of the sigmoid colon.

HEMATOLOGIC SYSTEM

Blood consists of plasma and cells suspended in the plasma. The plasma consists of water and dissolved proteins, electrolytes, and organic and inorganic substances. Blood cells include erythrocytes (RBCs), leukocytes (WBCs), and platelets (Figure 5-6). A variety of noninvasive and invasive laboratory and diagnostic tests are used to evaluate and monitor the hematologic system. Hematology reference ranges are listed in Table 5-4.

GENERAL LABORATORY TESTS
ABO Blood Typing.   The antigenic properties of blood are typed to avoid potentially lethal transfusion reactions. Blood types include A, B, AB, and O.

Blood Smear.   The blood smear is produced by smearing a drop of peripheral blood on a slide and examining the smear microscopically. The blood smear is used to

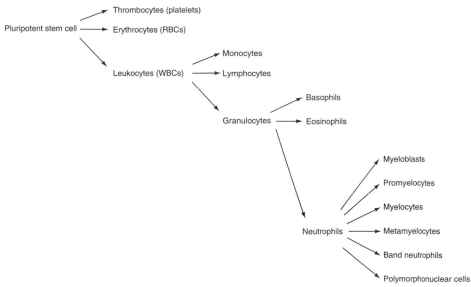

Figure 5-6
Cell Line Relationships.
All cell lines are derived from pluripotent stem cells.

TABLE 5-4

Adult Hematology Reference Laboratory Values

Index	Source	Reference Range
Bleeding time		2-9.5 min
Blood volume		8.5%-9.5% of body weight in kg
Erythrocyte count	WB	$4.15\text{-}4.9 \times 10^6/mm^3$
Erythrocyte sedimentation rate		
Female	WB	1-30 mm/hr
Male	WB	1-13 mm/hr
Ferritin	S	>20 ng/ml
Fibrin degradation products	S	<10 µg/ml
Folic acid	S	≥3.3 ng/ml
Hematocrit		
Female	WB	37%-48%
Male	WB	42%-52%
Hemoglobin		
Female	WB	12-16 g/dl
Male	WB	13-18 g/dl
Iron	S	50-150 µg/dl
Iron-binding capacity	S	250-410 µg/dl
Leukocyte count	WB	$4.3\text{-}10.8 \times 10^3/mm^3$
T lymphocytes	WB	74%-86% of circulating lymphocytes
B lymphocytes	WB	5%-25% of circulating lymphocytes
T4 lymphocytes (CD4)	WB	38%-52% of circulating lymphocytes
T8 lymphocytes (CD8)	WB	22%-36% of circulating lymphocytes
T4/T8 ratio		1.0:2.2
Mean corpuscular volume (MCV)	WB	$86\text{-}98 \ \mu m^3$
Mean corpuscular hemoglobin (MCH)	WB	28-33 pg/cell
Mean corpuscular hemoglobin concentration (MCHC)	WB	32-36 g/dl
Partial thromboplastin time, activated (aPTT)	P	24-37 sec
Platelet count	WB	$150\text{-}350 \times 10^3/mm^3$
Prothrombin time (PT)	P	8.8-11.6 sec
Red cell distribution width	WB	11.5%-14.5%
Reticulocyte count	WB	0.5%-2.5% of red cells
Thrombin time	P	Control ± 5 sec
Vitamin B_{12}	S	205-876 pg/ml

From Jordan CD et al: N Engl J Med 327:718-724, 1992; Sacher RA, McPherson RA: *Widmann's clinical interpretation of laboratory tests*, ed 11, Philadelphia, 2000, FA Davis; and Tilkian SM, Conover MB, Tilkian AG: *Clinical nursing implications of laboratory tests*, ed 5, St Louis, 1996, Mosby.
P, Plasma; S, serum; WB, whole blood.

obtain a WBC count and differential, to estimate the platelet count, and to evaluate RBC morphology.

Coagulation Tests. The common tests of coagulation include the bleeding time, PTT, PT, and thrombin time.

Activated Partial Thromboplastin Time. The activated partial thromboplastin time (aPTT) assesses the intrinsic clotting pathway (i.e., factors II, V, VIII, IX, X, XI, and XII). It is commonly used to monitor heparin therapy.

Bleeding Time. The bleeding time is the duration of bleeding after a standardized skin incision. It is used to evaluate platelet quantity and function.

Prothrombin Time. The PT is used to assess the extrinsic and common clotting pathways (i.e., factors II, V, VII, and X and fibrinogen). It is used to monitor warfarin therapy and to assess hepatic synthetic function. The international normalized ratio (INR) is a more standardized expression of PT that takes into account differences in reagent activity. It is calculated according to the equation $INR = (PT_{patient} \div PT_{control})^{ISI}$, where ISI is the International Sensitivity Index.

Thrombin Time. The thrombin time is used to evaluate the effect of heparin and thrombolytic drug therapy and coagulation abnormalities.

Complete Blood Count. The complete blood count (CBC) consists of the hemoglobin, hematocrit, RBC count, WBC count, mean corpuscular volume, mean corpuscular hemoglobin, and mean corpuscular hemoglobin concentration.

Crossmatching. Crossmatching determines compatibility between donor and recipient blood. Agglutination between the donor's RBCs and the recipient's serum indicates incompatibility.

Fibrinogen. Fibrinogen is increased in disseminated intravascular coagulation. It is used to evaluate bleeding disorders.

Fibrin Degradation Products. Fibrin degradation products (FDPs) are released when fibrin is broken down. They are assessed in the diagnosis and monitoring of disseminated intravascular coagulation.

Hemoglobin Electrophoresis. Immunoelectrophoresis uses electrophoretic separation and immunodiffusion to screen for the presence of abnormal proteins such as Bence Jones and myeloma proteins.

Serum Protein Electrophoresis. Serum protein electrophoresis (SPEP) is used to screen for serum protein abnormalities. The proteins (albumin, α_1 globulin, α_2 globulin, beta globulin, and gamma globulin) are identified by different migration patterns when subjected to an electric field.

LABORATORY TESTS BY SPECIFIC CELL TYPE

Platelets. Platelets initiate hemostasis. The risk of spontaneous bleeding is greatly increased if the platelet count is less than 20,000 cells/mm^3. The platelet count is sometimes estimated from the peripheral blood smear; it is considered adequate if the smear contains two to three platelets per field. The count may be performed manually or electronically and is a more accurate estimate of the number of platelets.

The platelet count and function are altered in a variety of diseases. The platelet count is decreased if the bone marrow fails to produce platelets (as in aplastic anemia, leukemia, and some viral infections) and by peripheral platelet destruction (as in idiopathic thrombocytopenic purpura, some collagen vascular diseases, thrombotic thrombocytopenic purpura, disseminated intravascular coagulation, and hemolytic uremic syndrome). The platelet count may be increased after splenectomy; in some myeloproliferative diseases, such as myelogenous leukemia and essential thrombocythemia; and in chronic inflammatory diseases, malignancy, and chronic infections. Platelet function is impaired by drugs such as aspirin, dipyridamole, and nonsteroidal antiinflammatory drugs and by disease states such as uremia, multiple myeloma, and severe liver disease.

Red Blood Cells

Carboxyhemoglobin. Carboxyhemoglobin forms in the presence of carbon monoxide (e.g., house fires, automobile exhaust). Carbon monoxide attaches to hemoglobin, rendering the hemoglobin incapable of carrying oxygen.

Coombs' Test. The Coombs' test is performed by using an antiserum containing antibodies that act to bridge antibody- or complement-coated RBCs. Agglutination occurs when the cells are bridged.

Direct Coombs' Test. The direct Coombs' test uses antibodies directed against human proteins (primarily immunoglobulin G [IgG] and complement [C_3]) to detect whether these proteins are attached to the surface of RBCs. The direct Coombs' test is used to differentiate between immunologic (e.g., autoimmune) and nonimmunologic (e.g., drug-induced) hemolytic anemias.

Indirect Coombs' Test. The indirect Coombs' test detects antibodies against human RBCs in the patient's serum. The indirect Coombs' test is used in crossmatching before transfusions.

Erythrocyte Sedimentation Rate. The erythrocyte sedimentation rate (ESR) is a nonspecific indicator of inflammation. This test measures the rate at which RBCs settle out of mixed venous blood. The settling rate, influenced by the shape of the RBC and the charges on the membrane, is used as a nonspecific marker of inflammatory and malignant disease.

Folate. Decreased serum folate levels are associated with megaloblastic anemias.

Hematocrit. The hematocrit is the number of RBCs in 100 ml of blood reported as a percentage. Reference ranges vary with age, gender, and elevation above sea level. The hematocrit is increased in vitamin B_{12} and folic acid deficiencies and is decreased in iron deficiency. The hematocrit is used to diagnose anemia and assess the patient's response to replacement therapy.

Hemoglobin. Hemoglobin is the oxygen-carrying RBC protein. Reference ranges vary with age, gender, and elevation above sea level. Hemoglobin is decreased in blood loss and iron deficiency anemia. Hemoglobin is used to diagnose anemia, assess the patient's response to replacement therapy, and estimate oxygen content.

Iron Metabolism

Ferritin. Serum ferritin does not contain iron but is in equilibrium with tissue ferritin, making it a useful indicator of tissue iron stores. It is used to diagnose iron deficiency anemia.

Iron. Serum iron levels are decreased in iron deficiency anemia, chronic infections, and some malignancies. Serum iron levels may be increased in iron poisoning and hemolysis.

Total Iron-Binding Capacity. The total iron-binding capacity (TIBC) test evaluates the capacity of transferrin to bind to iron. It is used to diagnose iron deficiency anemia and to monitor replacement therapy.

Transferrin Saturation. Transferrin is a specific iron transport protein. This test evaluates the percentage of total iron-binding protein saturated with iron. It is used to diagnose iron deficiency anemia and to monitor replacement therapy.

Red Blood Cell Appearance. The size, shape, and color of RBCs are influenced by many diseases. A variety of terms are used to describe the RBC appearance:

Acanthocytes. Acanthocytes, RBCs with long, thin, irregularly placed spines on the membrane, are associated with alcoholic cirrhosis and heparin therapy and may appear after splenectomy.

Anisocytosis. Anisocytosis, variably sized RBCs, is associated with early iron replacement therapy.

Burr Cells. Burr cells, RBCs with evenly distributed spicules on the membrane, are associated with uremia.

Elliptocytes. Elliptocytes, rod-shaped RBCs, are associated with sickle cell trait and thalassemia.

Hypochromia. Hypochromia is a decrease in the hemoglobin content of the RBCs. It produces pale RBCs and is associated with folic acid and vitamin B_{12} deficiency anemias.

Macrocytes. Macrocytes are larger-than-normal RBCs.

Microcytes. Microcytes are smaller-than-normal RBCs.

Normochromia. Normochromia describes normal RBC color.

Normocytes. Normocytes are normal-sized RBCs.

Ovalocytes. Ovalocytes, oval-shaped RBCs, are associated with microcytic and megaloblastic anemias.

Schistocytes. Schistocytes, RBC fragments, are associated with disseminated intravascular coagulation, prosthetic heart valves, uremia, and sickle cell anemia.

Spherocytes. Spherocytes, small, round RBCs, are associated with anemias and hemolytic transfusion reactions.

Stomatocytes. Stomatocytes, RBCs with central slitlike areas of pallor, are associated with neoplastic, liver, and cardiac disease.

Target Cells. Target cells, RBCs with dark centers surrounded by light rings, are associated with sickle cell anemia, iron deficiency, and liver disease; they also may occur after splenectomy.

Red Blood Cell Count. The RBC count is the number of RBCs per 1 ml of blood. It is used to diagnose anemias and to assess the patient's response to replacement therapy. It also serves as an indicator of chronic hypoxemia.

Red Blood Cell Inclusions. RBCs may contain abnormal material, known as *inclusions*.

Basophilic Stippling. Basophilic stippling is fine stippling associated with lead poisoning and some anemias.

Heinz Bodies. Heinz bodies, masses of denatured hemoglobin, are associated with severe oxidative stress and thalassemia.

Howell-Jolly Bodies. Howell-Jolly bodies, fragments of nuclear deoxyribonucleic acid (DNA) that appear as dark purple dots, may occur after splenectomy and also are associated with hemolytic and megaloblastic anemias.

Nucleated Red Blood Cells. Nucleated RBCs, less mature RBCs with nuclei, are associated with intense marrow erythropoietic activity.

Red Blood Cell Indices. The RBC indices consist of the mean cell volume, mean cell hemoglobin, and mean cell hemoglobin concentration. These indices are used to differentiate the type of anemia and to assess the patient's response to replacement drug therapy.

Mean Cell Hemoglobin. Mean cell hemoglobin (MCH) is the average RBC hemoglobin content. MCH is decreased in iron deficiency anemias and increased in folic acid and vitamin B_{12} deficiencies and hemolytic anemias.

Mean Cell Hemoglobin Concentration. Mean cell hemoglobin concentration (MCHC) is the amount of hemoglobin per volume of RBCs.

Mean Cell Volume. Mean cell volume (MCV) is the average volume of individual RBCs. MCV is decreased in iron deficiency anemias, thalassemias, and other chronic diseases (i.e., microcytic anemias). It is increased in folic acid and vitamin B_{12} deficiencies (i.e., macrocytic anemias).

Red Cell Distribution Width. The red cell distribution width (RDW) is a histogram of the distribution of RBC volumes as measured with automated equipment. It is used to diagnose anemias and to assess the patient's response to replacement therapy.

Reticulocytes. Reticulocytes are immature RBCs that contain residual ribonucleic acid (RNA) and protoporphyrin but no nucleus. The reticulocyte count is used to assess the response of the bone marrow to blood loss, hemolysis, and replacement therapy for the treatment of anemia. Healthy marrow produces and releases reticulocytes in response to the need for increased oxygen-carrying capacity.

Vitamin B_{12}. Decreased serum vitamin B_{12} levels are associated with megaloblastic anemias.

White Blood Cells. The three morphologically distinct types of WBCs include granulocytes (neutrophils, basophils, and eosinophils), monocytes, and lymphocytes. The WBC count and differential (the relative percentage and absolute numbers of each type of WBC) are used to diagnose a variety of diseases and to assess the patient's response to drug therapy.

Granulocytes

Eosinophils. Eosinophils are WBCs that contain numerous inflammatory mediators. The number of eosinophils is increased in parasitic infections and allergic reactions. Some neoplastic diseases, skin disorders, and collagen vascular diseases also may increase the number of circulating eosinophils.

Basophils. Basophils form heparin and have a role similar to that of mast cells in immediate hypersensitivity reactions. Basophils have insignificant phagocytic properties and do not increase in number as a result of infectious processes. The number of basophils may increase in chronic hypersensitivity states, systemic mast cell disease, and myeloproliferative diseases.

Neutrophils. Polymorphonuclear cells are mature WBCs. Their precursors, in order of increasing maturity, are myeloblasts, promyelocytes, myelocytes, metamyelocytes, and band neutrophils. A shift to the left in the differential WBC count means significant numbers of neutrophil precursors, such as bands, are present. Neutrophils are phagocytic cells that engulf and destroy bacteria. The number of neutrophils is increased in infections, tissue necrosis, inflammatory diseases, metabolic disorders, and some leukemias. The number of circulating neutrophils is increased by corticosteroids, exercise, and epinephrine, all of which induce the release of neutrophils from peripheral storage sites. The number of neutrophils is decreased in overwhelming infection and in some bacterial, viral, and protozoal infections. Marrow depressants, liver disease, and some collagen vascular diseases are associated with decreased numbers of neutrophils.

Lymphocytes. Lymphocytes, WBCs formed in lymphoid tissue throughout the body, provide humoral, cell-mediated, and cytotoxic immune responses and interact with antigens in the body. T lymphocytes, derived from the thymus, provide cell-mediated immunity; B lymphocytes, derived from the bone marrow, provide humoral immunity and produce antibodies. Null lymphocytes have neither T-cell nor B-cell characteristics. The lymphocyte count is increased in viral disease, bacterial diseases such as whooping cough, metabolic disease, and chronic inflammatory conditions. The lymphocyte count is decreased in immunodeficiency syndromes, severe illnesses, and diseases associated with abnormalities of the lymphatic circulatory system.

The two types of T lymphocytes include the T4 (helper) and T8 (suppressor) lymphocytes. T4 lymphocytes enhance the response of B cells. T4 lymphocytes are profoundly decreased in acquired immunodeficiency syndrome (AIDS). T8 lymphocytes may be increased in hepatitis B, acute mononucleosis, and cytomegaloviral infection. The T4-to-T8 lymphocyte ratio reverses in diseases associated with altered immunoregulatory function.

Monocytes. Monocytes, macrophage precursors, circulate briefly before entering body tissues, where they become macrophages. The monocyte count is increased in some infectious, granulomatous, and collagen vascular diseases.

DIAGNOSTIC PROCEDURE
Bone Marrow Aspiration. Bone marrow is obtained by penetrating the iliac crest or sternum with a large-bore needle and withdrawing a sample of the bone marrow. The sample is smeared on a slide and evaluated microscopically for cell-line precursors and iron stores. Bone marrow aspiration is used to diagnose anemias and leukemias.

IMMUNOLOGIC SYSTEM

A variety of laboratory tests and procedures are used to evaluate and monitor the immunologic system. Immunologic reference ranges are listed in Table 5-5.

LABORATORY TESTS
Autoantibodies. Autoantibodies are used in the monitoring and diagnosis of a variety of autoimmune diseases.[21,22]

Antineutrophil Cytoplasmic Antibodies. Antineutrophil cytoplasmic antibodies (ANCA) are autoantibodies against neutrophil granules and monocyte lysosomes. p-ANCA reactivity is associated with angiitis, rheumatoid arthritis, inflammatory bowel disease, and vasculitis. c-ANCA reactivity is associated with Wegener's granulomatosis.

Antinuclear Antibodies. Antinuclear antibodies (ANAs) often are associated with systemic lupus erythematosus (SLE), although they may be present in rheumatoid collagen diseases, mixed connective tissue disease, and systemic sclerosis. ANAs are reported as a titer and a pattern of cellular fluorescence. The patterns include the following:
1. *Homogenous*—diffuse fluorescence throughout the nucleus
2. *Ring*—nuclear border fluorescence
3. *Speckled*—speckled fluorescence throughout the nucleus
4. *Nucleolar*—fluorescence in the nucleolar area of the nucleus

TABLE 5-5

Adult Immunologic Laboratory Reference Values (Based on Serum Tests)

Index	Reference Range
Alpha₁-antitrypsin	85-213 mg/dl
Alpha-fetoprotein	<10 IU/ml
Antineutrophil cytoplasmic antibodies	Negative
Antinuclear antibodies	Negative at 1:8 dilution
Antinative DNA antibodies	Negative at 1:10 dilution
Antibodies to Sm	None
Antibodies to ribonucleoprotein (RNP)	None
Antibodies to SS-A (Ro)	None
Antibodies to SS-B (La)	None
Complement	
C_3	83-177 mg/dl
C_4	15-45 mg/dl
Total hemolytic (CH_{50})	150-250 U/ml
Rheumatoid factor	<30 IU/ml
Uric acid	
Female	2.3-6.6 mg/dl
Male	3.6-8.5 mg/dl

From Jordan DC et al: N Engl J Med 327:718-724, 1992; Sacher RA, McPherson RA: *Widmann's clinical interpretation of laboratory tests*, ed 11, Philadelphia, 2000, FA Davis; and Tilkian SM, Conover MB, Tilkian AG: *Clinical nursing implications of laboratory tests*, ed 5, St Louis, 1996, Mosby.

Anti-DNA Antibodies.   Anti-DNA antibodies are antibodies against double-stranded DNA (dsDNA) and single-stranded DNA (ssDNA). Anti-dsDNA antibodies often are found in patients with SLE.

Extractable Nuclear Antigens.   Antibodies may be present against specific extractable nuclear antigens (ENAs). These antigens include the Smith (Sm), ribonucleoprotein (RNP), SS-A (Ro), SS-B (La), Scl-70, and histone antigens. SLE is associated with high titers of anti-Sm antibodies. Mixed connective tissue disease and SLE are associated with high titers of anti-RNP antibodies. Systemic sclerosis and SLE are associated with high titers of anti-SS-A and anti-SS-B antibodies. Antibodies against histones may be found in patients with drug-induced SLE. Considerable overlap occurs among the diseases associated with these antibodies.

Rheumatoid Factor (RF).   Antibodies against IgG and IgM may be found in patients with rheumatoid arthritis.

Cold Agglutinins.   Cold agglutinins are antibodies that bind to the surface of RBCs.[23] Agglutination occurs when the blood sample is cooled. Cold agglutinins are associated with a variety of infections and inflammatory disorders.

Coombs' Test.   The Coombs' test uses an antiserum containing antibodies that bridge antibody- or complement-coated RBCs; bridging causes agglutination (clumping).

Direct Coombs' Test. The direct Coombs' test uses antibodies directed against human proteins (primarily IgG and C_3) to detect whether these proteins are attached to the surface of RBCs. The direct Coombs' test is used to differentiate between immunologic (e.g., autoimmune) and nonimmunologic (e.g., drug-induced) hemolytic anemias.

Indirect Coombs' Test. The indirect Coombs' test detects antibodies against human RBCs in the patient's serum. It is used in crossmatching before transfusion.

Complement. The total serum hemolytic complement (CH_{50}) test is used to screen the integrity of the complement system by testing in vitro the reaction of the patient's serum with presensitized sheep erythrocytes. CH_{50} levels decrease with increased autoimmune disease activity.

Complement Components 3 and 4. Components 3 and 4 (C_3 and C_4) of the complement system are normally found in relatively high quantities in the serum and are used to diagnose and monitor the progress of autoimmune disease activity.[24] C_3 and C_4 levels decrease with increased disease activity.

C-Reactive Protein. C-reactive protein, a nonspecific indicator of inflammation, is acutely elevated in rheumatoid arthritis, acute bacterial infections, and viral hepatitis. It also is sometimes used to differentiate between bacterial and viral meningitis.

Erythrocyte Sedimentation Rate. The ESR is a nonspecific indicator of inflammation. This test measures the rate at which RBCs settle out of mixed venous blood. The rate of settling is influenced by the shape of the RBCs and charges on the membrane. It is a nonspecific marker of inflammatory and malignant disease.

Immunoelectrophoresis. Immunoelectrophoresis uses electrophoretic separation and immunodiffusion techniques to separate proteins. It is used to screen for diseases associated with immunoglobulin abnormalities.

Immunoglobulin E. Serum immunoglobulin E (IgE) is elevated in patients with allergic disorders.

Lupus Anticoagulant. The lupus anticoagulant is a circulating immunoglobulin found in patients with autoimmune disease. It prolongs in vitro clotting time by inhibiting phospholipid interactions but is not associated with an increased risk of bleeding in vivo.

Organ-Specific Autoantibodies. Autoantibodies directed against antigens unique to specific organs may be associated with diseases. For example, antibodies may be detected against the thyroid (thyroiditis), RBC membranes (autoimmune hemolytic anemia), platelet membranes (immune thrombocytopenic purpura), glomerular basement membranes (Goodpasture's disease and glomerulonephritis), intrinsic factor (pernicious anemia), and the acetylcholine receptor (myasthenia gravis).

Protein Electrophoresis. Serum protein electrophoresis is used to screen for serum protein abnormalities. The proteins (albumin, α_1 globulin, α_2 globulin, beta globulin, and gamma globulin) are separated by different migration patterns they follow when subjected to an electric field. This test is used in the diagnosis of diseases associated with immunoglobulin abnormalities.

Uric Acid.   Uric acid is the end product of purine metabolism. Low serum levels are associated with Wilson's disease and some malabsorption syndromes. High levels are associated with rapid cellular destruction (as in chemotherapy or malignancies) and disorders of metabolism such as gout.

Venereal Disease Research Laboratory Test.   The Venereal Disease Research Laboratory (VDRL) test, used to diagnose syphilis, is sometimes falsely positive in connective tissue disease.

DIAGNOSTIC PROCEDURES
Anergy Panel.   An anergy panel is used to test the patient's reactivity to a variety of antigens (purified protein derivative antigen, mumps antigen, *Streptococcus* antigen, *Candida*, *Trichophyton* antigen, histoplasmin). The antigens are injected intradermally, and the skin is evaluated for redness and swelling at the injection site. Response to one or more of the antigens indicates a responsive immune system. Response to a specific antigen indicates that the patient has antibodies to a specific antigen.

Scratch or Patch Testing.   Scratch testing is used to evaluate patient sensitivity to specific allergens.[25] Each allergen is applied to the skin by scratching the skin. The skin is then evaluated for swelling and redness.

INFECTIOUS DISEASE

A variety of laboratory and diagnostic tests and procedures are used to diagnose infectious disease and to monitor the patient's response to drug therapy.

LABORATORY TESTS
Acid-Fast Stain.   The acid-fast stain is used to screen for the presence of *Mycobacterium, Nocardia,* and *Legionella* species in body tissues and fluids. Some oocysts, such as *Cryptosporidium,* can be detected with the acid-fast stain.

Cerebrospinal Fluid Analysis.   The cerebrospinal fluid is analyzed for the presence and quantity of RBCs, WBCs, glucose, and protein. If indicated, stains (Gram's stain and acid-fast stain) and potassium hydroxide and India ink preparations are used to evaluate the fluid. Normally, the cerebrospinal fluid is clear, without blood or organisms. The cerebrospinal fluid glucose is normally about two-thirds the serum blood glucose. Viral meningitis is characterized by a negative Gram's stain and normal protein and glucose. Fungal and tuberculous meningitis is characterized by a negative Gram's stain, normal protein, and low glucose. Bacterial meningitis is characterized by cloudy cerebrospinal fluid, increased WBCs, elevated protein, and frequently a positive Gram's stain.

Cold Agglutinins.   Cold agglutinins are antibodies that bind to the surface of RBCs and agglutinate when the blood sample is cooled. About 50% of patients with *Mycoplasma pneumoniae* have cold agglutinin titers.

C-Reactive Protein.   C-reactive protein, a nonspecific indicator of inflammation, is acutely elevated in rheumatoid arthritis, acute bacterial infections, and viral hepatitis. It is sometimes used to differentiate between bacterial and viral meningitis.

Culture and Sensitivity Testing.   Cultures of body fluids and tissues identify specific infecting organisms. In vitro testing is used to determine antibiotic susceptibilities.

Cytotoxicity Toxin Assays.   The presence of some infectious microorganisms is identified by the presence of specific toxins produced by them rather than by identification of the organism itself. For example, *Clostridium difficile* is detected by the presence of a toxin in the stool.

Gram's Stain.   The Gram's stain is used to evaluate a body fluid or specimen for the presence of microorganisms. The organisms are characterized according to their gram-positive or gram-negative characteristics, morphology (e.g., cocci, rod), and other characteristics (e.g., chain or cluster formation).

India Ink Preparation.   The India ink preparation is used to detect *Cryptococcus neoformans* in a variety of body fluids. The carbons in India ink are unable to penetrate the organism, enabling the microscopic identification of the organism by its lack of staining.

Minimal Bactericidal Concentration.   The minimal bactericidal concentration (MBC) is the lowest antibiotic concentration that kills at least 99.9% of the bacteria in the original inoculum. It is used to determine the susceptibility of the organism to antibiotics.

Minimum Inhibitory Concentration.   The minimum inhibitory concentration (MIC) is the lowest antibiotic concentration that completely inhibits the visible growth of a microorganism. It is used to determine the susceptibility of the organism to antibiotics.

Potassium Hydroxide Preparation.   Potassium hydroxide (KOH) 10% to 20% is used to detect fungi in body fluids and skin scrapings.

Rapid Plasma Reagin Test.   The rapid plasma reagin (RPR) test is used to screen for syphilis. It tests for antibodies against antigens from damaged host cells.

Serologic Tests.   Serologic tests are used to identify an antigen or antibody to help diagnose infectious disease and to monitor the immunologic response to the microorganism.[26] Acute-phase titers and convalescent titers are sometimes compared. Example of serologic tests include the antistreptolysin-O (ASO) titer, cold agglutinin titers, cryptococcal titers, and hepatitis viral serology.

Venereal Disease Research Laboratory Test.   The VDRL test, used to diagnose syphilis and neurosyphilis, tests for antibodies against antigens from damaged host cells. The VDRL test is not as sensitive as the RPR test.

Wet Mounts.   Wet mounts of body fluid specimens are examined microscopically for the presence of parasites and fungi.

White Blood Cell Count and Differential. The WBC count is often elevated in patients with bacterial and viral infections. A left shift (increased bands and segmented neutrophils) indicates a bacterial infection. The lymphocyte count may be elevated in viral infections. The eosinophil count may be elevated in parasitic infections. Elderly patients and those with impaired immune systems or very severe infectious diseases may not be able to mount a white cell response to infection.

NEUROLOGIC SYSTEM

The neurologic system is evaluated with several highly specialized diagnostic tests and procedures.

DIAGNOSTIC PROCEDURES

Cold Calorics. Cold calorics assesses brainstem function in comatose patients. The intact external auditory canal is filled with ice-cold water. Both eyes move toward the cold ear and then snap back to the center if brainstem function is normal.

Edrophonium (Tensilon) Test. The edrophonium test is used to diagnosis myasthenia gravis and to determine whether the maintenance acetylcholinesterase inhibitor dosage is appropriate. Edrophonium is administered parenterally, and the muscle strength of the patient is evaluated subjectively.

Electroencephalography. The electroencephalograph (EEG) records the electrical activity of the brain from electrodes attached to the scalp. It is used to diagnose seizures and to assess the patient's response to drug therapy.

Electromyography. Electromyography (EMG) evaluates muscle action potential from needles inserted into the muscle. It is used to diagnose muscle disease and to evaluate the patient's response to therapy.

Peripheral Nerve Stimulation. Peripheral nerve stimulation assesses depth of neuromuscular blockade. Four supramaximal ("Train-of-Four") electrical impulses are applied to a peripheral nerve (ulnar, posterior tibial, facial, or peroneal); the number of resultant twitches is counted. No twitches, one twitch, two twitches, three twitches, and four twitches indicate 100%, 90%, 75%, and 50% blockade, respectively.

Nerve Conduction Studies. The rate of nerve conduction is evaluated by stimulating the nerve and recording the rate of conduction to electrodes placed over the muscle. Nerve conduction studies are used to diagnose nerve injuries and neuromuscular disease.

NUTRITIONAL ASSESSMENT

Numerous parameters in addition to height and weight are used to assess the nutritional status of a patient and to monitor the patient's response to supplemental or total nutritional replacement therapy.[27-29] Nutritional assessment references ranges are listed in Table 5-6.

TABLE 5-6

Adult Nutritional Laboratory Reference Values

Index	Source	Reference Range
Alanine aminotransferase (ALT)		
Female	S	7-30 U/L
Male	S	10-55 U/L
Aspartate aminotransferase (AST)		
Female	S	9-25 U/L
Male	S	10-40 U/L
Bilirubin		
Direct	S	Up to 0.4 mg/dl
Total	S	Up to 1 mg/dl
Blood urea nitrogen	S	8-25 mg/dl
Calcium	S	8.5-10.5 mg/dl
Glucose (fasting)	P	70-110 mg/dl
Hemoglobin		
Female	WB	12-16 g/dl
Male	WB	13-18 g/dl
Iron	S	50-150 µg/dl
Magnesium	S	1.5-2.0 mEq/L
Partial thromboplastin time, activated (aPTT)	P	24-37 sec
Phosphorus, inorganic	S	2.6-4.5 mg/dl
Protein		
Albumin	S	3.1-4.3 g/dl
Total	S	6-8 g/dl (60-80 g/L)
Total	U	<165 mg/day
Transferrin saturation	S	20%-45%

From Jordan CD et al: N Engl J Med 327:718-724, 1992; Sacher RA, McPherson RA: Widmann's clinical interpretation of laboratory tests, ed 11, Philadelphia, 2000, FA Davis; and Tilkian SM, Conover MB, Tilkian AG: Clinical nursing implications of laboratory tests, ed 5, St Louis, 1996, Mosby.
P, Plasma; S, serum; U, urine; WB, whole blood.

LABORATORY TESTS

Albumin.   Serum albumin is an indicator of visceral protein reserves and nutritional status. Protein malnutrition is associated with a serum albumin level of less than 3.5 mg/dl if liver function is normal.

Bilirubin.   Conjugation of bilirubin requires energy; starvation may cause mild hyperbilirubinemia.

Calcium.   Decreased serum albumin decreases total calcium. However, the serum calcium does not reflect total body stores.

Creatinine.   The 24-hour urinary excretion of creatinine is used to estimate muscle catabolism. Although serum creatinine is not a useful indicator of nutritional status, very low serum creatinine levels may reflect poor nutritional status.

Glucose.   Blood glucose is monitored during nutritional supplementation or total nutritional replacement therapy to assess overall metabolic balance. It is not a useful indicator of nutritional status.

Immunologic Status.   Malnutrition may be associated with altered immunologic status. Lymphocyte production may be diminished, resulting in a decreased total lymphocyte count. Patients may not be able to mount an immunologic response to skin test antigens.

Magnesium.   Decreased serum albumin levels decrease total magnesium. However, the serum magnesium does not reflect total body stores.

Partial Thromboplastin Time.   Poor nutritional status may be associated with inadequate intake of vitamin K, resulting in a deficiency of vitamin K–dependent clotting factors and prolonged clotting time.

Phosphorus.   Phosphorus is a metabolic cofactor and intermediate. Refeeding hypophosphatemia may occur in patients with low levels of phosphorus who receive nutritional supplementation or total nutritional replacement therapy.

Transaminases.   Starvation compromises cellular membrane integrity and may be associated with increased transaminases (AST and ALT).

Transferrin.   Transferrin is an iron transport protein with a shorter half-life than albumin (1 week versus 3 weeks). Serum transferrin responds more quickly to changes in nutritional status than does albumin and is a useful indicator of nutritional status.

Urea Nitrogen, Blood.   Blood urea nitrogen (BUN) is a useful indicator of protein breakdown.

DIAGNOSTIC PROCEDURES
Anthropometrics.   Comparative body measurements assess nutritional status. Parameters such as skin-fold thickness of the upper portion of the nondominant arm, midupper arm circumference (MUAC), and arm muscle circumference (AMC) are assessed. In general, a 20% to 40% decrease compared with normal values is associated with moderate malnutrition. A greater than 40% decrease is associated with severe malnutrition.

RENAL SYSTEM

A variety of laboratory tests are used to diagnose the renal system and monitor the patient's response to drug therapy. Renal system reference ranges are listed in Table 5-7.

LABORATORY TESTS
Arterial Blood Gas.   The arterial blood gas assesses acid-base balance and ventilation. It is used to diagnose acid-base disturbances and to monitor the patient's response to drug and nondrug interventions.

   Arterial pH.   The arterial pH is a quantitative measure of the degree of acidity or alkalinity of the arterial blood.

TABLE 5-7

Adult Renal and Mineral Laboratory Reference Values

Index	Source	Reference Range
Arterial blood gas		
pH	WB	7.35-7.45
P_{CO_2}	WB	35-45 mm Hg
P_{O_2}	WB	75-100 mm Hg
Bicarbonate	WB	22-26 mEq/L
Oxygen saturation	WB	96%-100%
Base excess	WB	−2 to +2
Calcium, ionized	S	4.6-5.1 mg/dl
Calcium, total	S	8.5-10.5 mg/dl
Carbon dioxide content	S	24-30.9 mEq/L
Chloride	S	100-108 mEq/L
Magnesium	S	1.5-2.0 mEq/L
Phosphorus	S	2.6-4.5 mg/dl
Potassium	S	3.5-5.0 mEq/L
Sodium	S	135-145 mEq/L
Specific gravity	U	1.001-1.030
Urine pH	U	4.8-7.8

From Jordan CD et al: N Engl J Med 327:718-724, 1992; Sacher RA, McPherson RA: Widmann's clinical interpretation of laboratory tests, ed 11, Philadelphia, 2000, FA Davis; and Tilkian SM, Conover MB, Tilkian AG: Clinical nursing implications of laboratory tests, ed 5, St Louis, 1996, Mosby.
S, Serum; U, urine; WB, whole blood.

Base Excess.   Base excess (BE) is a quantitative measurement of the combined buffering capacity of all body buffering systems, including the bicarbonate system and hemoglobin.

Bicarbonate.   The bicarbonate is a quantitative measure of net bicarbonate production and elimination.

Carbon Dioxide Tension.   The partial pressure of dissolved carbon dioxide (Pa_{CO_2}) is a quantitative measure of net carbon dioxide production and elimination.

Oxygen Saturation.   The oxygen saturation of the blood (Sa_{O_2}) is a quantitative measurement of the percentage of hemoglobin combined with oxygen. It can be measured noninvasively with pulse oximetry.[30]

Oxygen Tension.   The partial pressure of oxygen dissolved in the blood (P_{O_2}) is a quantitative measure of oxygen concentration.

Creatinine.   Creatinine, filtered by glomeruli, is a useful indicator of renal function.

Electrolytes and Minerals.   Serum electrolytes and minerals that are useful when assessing the renal system include calcium, chloride, magnesium, phosphorus, potassium, and sodium. However, the serum concentration of these electrolytes and minerals is variable and does not reflect total body stores.

Calcium (Ionized).   Ionized (free) calcium is the physiologic active portion of total serum calcium. Ionized calcium is used to assess calcium status in patients with or at risk of secondary hyperparathyroidism (e.g., renal failure) and in patients with hypomagnesemia, sepsis, and pancreatitis.

Calcium (Total).   Approximately 40% of serum calcium is bound to albumin in a ratio of 0.8 mg/dl of calcium per 1.0 g/dl albumin. Approximately 15% of serum calcium is bound to albumin; the remaining 45% of serum calcium is unbound ionized (free) calcium. Total serum calcium, the sum of bound and free calcium, is used to assess calcium metabolism and to screen for and evaluate the response to therapy in bone tumors, primary and secondary hyperparathyroidism and hypoparathyroidism, renal failure, and acute pancreatitis.

Chloride.   Chloride is an extracellular electrolyte. Serum chloride is increased in renal tubular acidosis and primary hyperparathyroidism. It is decreased by the administration of drugs such as thiazide, loop diuretics, and corticosteroids.

Magnesium.   Magnesium is an intracellular electrolyte. Serum magnesium is used in the assessment of magnesium deficiency and for monitoring of replacement therapy.

Phosphorus.   Phosphorus is present in bone (about 85% of the total) and skeletal muscle (about 10% of the total). The serum phosphorus concentration is always in a 1:1 ratio with the serum calcium concentration. Serum phosphorus is used in the diagnosis of hypoparathyroidism and the assessment of bone metabolism.

Potassium.   Potassium is an intracellular electrolyte. The serum concentration is sensitive to changes in acid-base status. Serum potassium is increased in acidosis, dehydration, and renal insufficiency and with the administration of some drugs, such as spironolactone. It is decreased in overhydration and alkalosis and with the administration of drugs such as corticosteroids, amphotericin, and lithium carbonate.

Sodium.   Sodium is an extracellular electrolyte used to assess water and sodium balance. Serum sodium is increased in dehydration. It is decreased in Addison's disease and by diuretic administration, dilution in ascites, congestive heart failure, renal insufficiency, and excessive water intake.

Gram's Stain and Culture.   Normal urine contains no bacteria or yeasts. Bacteria are present in urinary tract infections and pyelonephritis. The Gram's stain and culture identify the cause of the infection and aid in monitoring the patient's response to drug therapy. Yeasts are found in the immunocompromised host and sometimes are associated with broad-spectrum antibiotic therapy.

Osmolality.   The urine and serum osmolalities are measured and compared to assess the kidneys' ability to concentrate the urine. The normal urine-to-serum osmolality ratio is 1:3. Ratios less than 1:1 indicate distal tubular disease. Ratios greater than 1:1 indicate glomerular disease.

Urea Nitrogen, Blood.   BUN, the end product of protein metabolism, is excreted by glomerular filtration. Although it is used as an indicator of renal function, it is less reliable than the serum creatinine because some of the urea diffuses back into the renal tubular cells after filtration. In addition, liver function and protein intake influence the production of BUN.

Urinary Sodium.   The urinary sodium is used to differentiate between renal failure from prerenal causes (e.g., dehydration) and from parenchymal renal insufficiency. In renal disease the kidneys are unable to conserve sodium, resulting in elevated urine sodium levels. Urinary sodium also is used to diagnose the syndrome of inappropriate antidiuretic hormone secretion (SIADH); in SIADH the serum sodium is low but the urine sodium is elevated.

Urine Toxicology.   Urinalysis is used to detect the presence of drugs in patients with suspected drug overdoses, patients experiencing altered mental status, and patients in drug rehabilitation programs.

Urinalysis.   Urinalysis is used to screen for renal and nonrenal disease and to monitor the patient's response to drug and nondrug therapy.[31,32] The urinalysis consists of macroscopic assessment, chemical screening by dipstick, and microscopic assessment of the urine sediment. Quantitative analyses are performed when indicated.

Dipstick Screening.   Multiple-reagent strips are used to determine the urinary pH and specific gravity and to screen for the presence of bilirubin, blood, glucose, ketones, leukocyte esterase, nitrites, pH, protein, and urobilinogen.

Bilirubin.   Bilirubin is not normally present in the urine. It is excreted in the urine in the presence of severe liver disease or obstructive biliary disease. The urine appears dark yellow to brown if bilirubin is present.

Blood.   Blood is not normally present in the urine. The urine may be visibly bloody, or blood may be found on microscopic or dipstick examination. A variety of renal and nonrenal diseases, including urinary tract infections, renal stones, sickle cell disease, glomerulonephritis, and malignant hypertension, are associated with blood in the urine.

Glucose.   Glucose is not normally present in the urine. Urine glucose may be present in diabetes mellitus.

Ketones.   Ketones are not normally present in the urine. Urinary ketones may be present before serum ketones are detectable in diabetic ketoacidosis and may be found in patients who are dieting or are malnourished.

Leukocyte Esterase.   Leukocyte esterase is not normally present in the urine. This enzyme is present in WBCs and may be found in the urine during urinary tract and vaginal infections.

Nitrites.   Nitrites are not normally present in the urine. *Escherichia coli* converts dietary nitrates to nitrites. Urinary nitrites are associated with *E. coli* urinary tract infections but may only be found if the urine is retained in the bladder for at least 4 hours.

pH.   The urinary pH reflects the overall acid-base balance of the body and the kidneys' ability to handle acids and bases. The formation of kidney stones is pH dependent. An alkaline pH (pH >7.0) is commonly associated with the presence of urea-splitting organisms such as *Proteus mirabilis.*

Protein.   Small amounts of protein are normally present in the urine (as much as 0.5 g/day). Urinary protein is increased in a variety of renal diseases.

Specific Gravity.   The specific gravity reflects the kidneys' ability to concentrate urine and the overall state of hydration. The greater the concentration of the urine is, the higher the specific gravity is.

Urobilinogen.   Urobilinogen is not normally present in the urine. It may be excreted in the urine in the presence of severe liver disease or obstructive biliary disease.

Macroscopic Assessment

Color.   Freshly voided urine is normally pale yellow. Normal urine may range in color from nearly colorless if very dilute to orange if very concentrated.

Turbidity.   Freshly voided urine is normally clear. The urine is turbid if bacteria, WBCs, RBCs, yeast, or crystals are present.

Microscopic Assessment.   The microscopic evaluation assesses the urinary sediment obtained by centrifugation for a variety of casts, cells, and crystals.

Casts.   Urinary casts, sometimes known as the *poor man's renal biopsy,* are objects formed and molded within renal tubules. Casts are cylindrical and composed mostly of protein and cells. They may be convoluted (spiral) if formed in distal convoluted tubules, broad if formed in dilated collecting ducts, and narrow if formed in narrow lumens.

Bile casts.   Bile casts are acellular casts that contain bile. They are associated with liver disease.

Granular casts.   Granular casts are acellular casts that have a granular appearance. They are associated with renal and viral disease and exercise.

Hemoglobin casts.   Hemoglobin casts are acellular casts that contain hemoglobin. They are associated with hemolytic anemias.

Hyaline casts.   Hyaline casts are acellular casts that consist of a protein matrix. An occasional hyaline cast may normally be present; however, the number of hyaline casts increases with renal disease.

Mixed cellular casts.   Mixed cellular casts may contain RBCs, WBCs, and renal tubular epithelial cells. These casts are associated with mixed tubular and interstitial renal diseases.

Red blood cell casts.   RBC casts are formed if the glomerular basement membrane is damaged. They may be found in acute and focal glomerulonephritis, lupus nephritis, and trauma.

Renal tubular epithelial cell casts.   Renal tubular epithelial cell casts are found in diseases such as hepatitis and cytomegaloviral infection associated with tubular epithelial destruction.

Waxy casts.   Waxy casts are acellular casts formed by the breakdown of cellular casts. They are associated with chronic renal disease.

White blood cell casts.   WBC casts are associated with interstitial renal inflammation and are found in pyelonephritis.

Cells

Red blood cells.   Normally, as many as two RBCs per high-power field may be present in the urine. The number of RBCs in the urine increases with urinary tract infections, stones, and tumors and with strenuous exercise.

Renal tubular epithelial cells.   Renal tubular epithelial cells, shed from the renal tubules, are normally present in the urine.

Squamous epithelial cells.   Squamous epithelial cells are normally present in the urine. They are shed from the urethra and vagina.

White blood cells.   Normally, as many as five neutrophils per high-power field may be found in the urine. The number of WBCs in the urine increases with renal and urinary tract disease and strenuous exercise.

Crystals.   Crystals are found in acidic and alkalotic urine. Amorphous phosphate crystals and triple phosphate crystals are normally present in alkaline urine. Amorphous urate crystals, calcium oxalate, and uric acid crystals are normally present in acidic urine. A variety of pathologic crystals may be found in alkaline urine.

Bilirubin crystals.   Bilirubin crystals are reddish brown needles, plates, and cubes associated with jaundice and bilirubinemia.

Cholesterol crystals.   Cholesterol crystals are flat plates with notched corners associated with the nephrotic syndromes.

Cysteine crystals.   Cysteine crystals are hexagonal plates associated with congenital cystinuria.

Leucine crystals.   Leucine crystals are round, oily-appearing crystals associated with severe hepatic disease.

Tyrosine crystals.   Tyrosine crystals are fine needles grouped in sheaves that are associated with severe hepatic disease.

DIAGNOSTIC PROCEDURES

Intravenous Pyelogram.   The intravenous pyelogram (IVP) is a test used to visualize the entire urinary tract.[33] A parenteral contrast medium cleared by glomerular filtration is used to detect ureteral obstruction, masses, tumors, and cysts.

Retrograde Pyelography.   Retrograde pyelography is used to visualize the urine-collecting systems independent of renal function. Contrast media are instilled through a catheter placed in the bladder.

RESPIRATORY SYSTEM

A variety of laboratory tests and diagnostic procedures are used to diagnose respiratory diseases and to monitor the patient's response to drug therapy.

LABORATORY TESTS

Arterial Blood Gas.   The arterial blood gas is used to assess the acid-base balance and level of ventilation, to diagnose acid-base disturbances, and to monitor the patient's response to drug and nondrug interventions. Refer to pages 133-134 for a discussion of the components of the arterial blood gas.

Sputum Analysis.   Sputum analysis is used to screen for disease and to monitor the patient's response to drug and nondrug therapy. It consists of macroscopic and microscopic assessments.

Macroscopic Assessment

Color.   The mucus is normally mucoid and clear. Purulent sputum contains pus and is associated with bacterial infection. Yellow sputum is indicative of inflammation. Uniformly rusty-appearing purulent sputum is indicative of *Pneumococcal pneumoniae* pneumonia. Bright red streaks in viscid sputum is indicative of *Klebsiella pneumoniae* pneumonia. Greenish black sputum is indicative of gram-negative bacilli infection.

Odor.   Normal sputum is odorless. Foul-smelling sputum is indicative of a bacterial infection.

Viscosity.   Normal sputum is thin and watery. Asthmatic patients have a very thick, sticky, tenacious sputum.

Volume.   Very little sputum is produced normally. The volume of sputum is increased in a variety of diseases, including bronchitis, pneumonia, and tuberculosis.

Microscopic Assessment

Charcot-Leyden Crystals.   Charcot-Leyden crystals are elongated double pyramid-shaped masses of eosinophils associated with asthma.

Curschmann's Spirals.   Curschmann's spirals are casts of small bronchi present in diseases associated with bronchial obstruction, such as asthma.

Eosinophils.   Eosinophils are present in asthma and other hypersensitivity disorders.

Neutrophils.   Neutrophils are found in bacterial and fungal pneumonia and chronic bronchitis.

DIAGNOSTIC PROCEDURES

Bronchoscopy.   Bronchoscopy is used to visualize the tracheobronchial tree. A flexible bronchoscope is introduced into the tracheobronchial tree through the nose, mouth, or endotracheal or tracheotomy tube. Samples of fluid and tissue may be obtained for Gram's stain, culture, and cytologic examination.[34]

Chest Radiography.   Chest x-ray films (see Figure 5-3) aid in the diagnosis of pulmonary and cardiac disease and the assessment of the patient's response to drug and nondrug interventions.[35]

Pulmonary Function Testing.   Pulmonary function testing is used to diagnose pulmonary disease, to monitor progression of disease, to predict response to bronchodilators, and to monitor the patient's response to drug and nondrug therapy. Pulmonary function testing is performed using a spirometer or body plethysmography. A spirometer detects and records changes in lung volume and flow. Body plethysmography detects changes in intrathoracic pressure and volume. Normal values vary with age, gender, height, and weight. In general, decreases of 20% or more from predicted values are considered significant.

Carbon Monoxide Diffusing Capacity.   The carbon monoxide diffusing capacity (D_{LCO}) test is a noninvasive test of lung function. It is an index of the surface area available for gas exchange and is decreased in emphysema, alveolar inflammation, and pulmonary fibrosis.

Forced Expiratory Volume in 1 Second.   The forced expiratory volume in 1 second (FEV_1) is the volume of air (in liters) exhaled during forced exhalation after maximal inspiration. Normally, at least 80% of the forced vital capacity (FVC) is exhaled in the first second. The FEV_1 is used with the FVC to differentiate between obstructive ($FEV_1/FVC < 80\%$) and restrictive (reduced FEV_1 and FVC but normal FEV_1/FVC relationship) lung disease. An FEV_1 of less than 1 L indicates significant lung disease.

Forced Vital Capacity.   The FVC is the volume of air (in liters) blown out of the lungs during forced exhalation after maximal inspiration. It is used with the FEV_1 to differentiate between obstructive and restrictive lung disease (see preceding FEV_1 discussion).

Peak Expiratory Flow Rate.   The peak expiratory flow rate (PEFR) measures the forced expiratory flow in liters per minute. It is used to monitor the progression and response to therapy of patients with bronchospastic diseases such as asthma. Asthmatic patients monitor their PEFR at home with inexpensive handheld peak flowmeters. PEFR variability of greater than 30% indicates moderate to severe persistent asthma.

Residual Volume.   The residual volume (RV) is the volume of air remaining in the lungs after forced expiration. It is measured with body plethysmography. RVs are increased in diseases characterized by small airway obstruction.

Tidal Volume.   The tidal volume (V_T) is the volume of air inspired or expired with normal breathing.

Pulse Oximetry.   Pulse oximetry is a noninvasive, transcutaneous technique used to assess oxygen saturation.

Quantitative Pilocarpine Iontophoresis (Sweat Test).   The concentration of sodium in sweat is measured after stimulation of the sweat glands with topical pilocarpine; low-voltage current is applied to aid in the absorption of the pilocarpine. The sweat test is used in the diagnosis of cystic fibrosis.

Ventilation/Perfusion Scanning. Ventilation/perfusion ($\dot{V}/\dot{Q}$) scanning is used to compare ventilation and perfusion. Images of the airways taken after the inhalation of radiolabeled tracers are compared with images of the pulmonary vasculature taken after the injection of contrast agents. Normally, ventilated and perfused areas match. This test is commonly used to identify pulmonary emboli.

SEROUS BODY FLUIDS

A variety of laboratory and diagnostic tests are used to evaluate serous body fluids. Pleural, pericardial, peritoneal, and synovial body fluids are examined to determine the cause (infectious, malignant, or inflammatory) of disease and the patient's response to drug and nondrug treatment. Exudates occur as a result of direct membrane and capillary damage; transudates occur when fluid leaks from blood vessels.

LABORATORY AND DIAGNOSTIC TESTS

Serous fluids are analyzed for gross appearance, specific gravity, cell counts and differential cell counts, protein, LDH, and cytology. Immunologic assays and cultures may be performed if indicated. Exudates typically have a cloudy appearance and greater specific gravity, protein, LDH, and cell counts than do transudates. The fluid-to-serum protein and fluid-to-serum LDH ratios are greater in exudates than in transudates.

In addition to the tests just described, synovial fluid may be evaluated for the presence and type of crystals.[36] Crystals are characterized by shape, birefringence in polarized light, and location (intracellular or extracellular). Two types of crystals may be found in synovial fluid.

Calcium Pyrophosphate Crystals. Calcium pyrophosphate crystals may be rod-shaped, needle-shaped, or rhombic. They have positive birefringence and are found intracellularly and extracellularly. They are associated with pseudogout.

Monosodium Urate Crystals. Monosodium urate crystals are needle-shaped, have negative birefringence, and are found intracellularly and extracellularly. They are associated with gout.

SELF-ASSESSMENT QUESTIONS

1. Which one of the following is a noninvasive test or procedure?
   a. Venipuncture
   b. Angiography
   c. Paracentesis
   d. Ultrasonography
   e. Radionuclide studies

2. Which one of the following procedures uses external magnetic fields to produce finely detailed images?
   a. CT
   b. MRI
   c. PET
   d. SPECT
   e. Doppler echography

3. A patient is found to have an elevated CK-MB, an elevated LDH_1 and a "flipped" LDH ratio. These results are consistent with a diagnosis of which of the following?
   a. Myocardial infarction
   b. Pneumonia
   c. Renal failure
   d. Cerebrovascular accident
   e. Liver failure

4. Radionuclide angiocardiography is also known as which of the following?
   a. Electrocardiography
   b. Lymphoscintigraphy
   c. Multiple gated acquisition scanning
   d. Echocardiography
   e. Electrophysiology

5. Metyrapone does which of the following?
   a. Stimulates cortisol synthesis
   b. Inhibits production of antidiuretic hormone
   c. Inhibits production of vanillylmandelic acid
   d. Increases urine aldosterone
   e. Inhibits cortisol synthesis

6. Which one of the following tests is used to assess hepatic synthetic function?
   a. Lactic dehydrogenase
   b. Serum albumin
   c. Aspartate aminotransferase
   d. Gamma glutamyl transpeptidase
   e. Total bilirubin

7. A schistocyte is which of the following?
   a. A red blood cell fragment
   b. A red blood cell with a dark center surrounded by a light ring
   c. A red blood cell shaped like a rod
   d. A red blood cell with evenly distributed spicules
   e. A red blood cell with fragments of nuclear DNA

8. Which one of the following is a laboratory test for fungal skin infections?
   a. Rapid plasma reagin test
   b. Venereal Disease Research Laboratory test
   c. Potassium hydroxide preparation
   d. White blood cell count with differential
   e. Cold agglutinin titer

9. Which one of the following is a quantitative measure of combined body buffering systems?
   a. P_{CO_2}
   b. Serum bicarbonate
   c. Oxygen saturation
   d. Base excess
   e. Serum creatinine

10. The macroscopic evaluation of sputum includes all of the following *except:*
    a. Color
    b. Viscosity
    c. Volume
    d. Odor
    e. Gram's stain

References

1. Jordan CD et al: Normal reference laboratory values, N Engl J Med 327:718-724, 1992.
2. Sacher RA, McPherson RA: Widmann's clinical interpretation of laboratory tests, ed 11, Philadelphia, 2000, FA Davis.
3. Tilkian SM, Conover MB, Tilkian AG: Clinical nursing implications of laboratory tests, ed 5, St Louis, 1996, Mosby.
4. Marshall T, Williams J, Williams KM: Electrophoresis of serum isoenzymes and proteins following acute myocardial infarction, J Chromatogr 569:323-345, 1991.
5. Technology Subcommittee of the Working Group on Critical Care: Hemodynamic monitoring: a technology assessment, Can Med Assoc J 145:114-121, 1991.
6. Taylor BC, Sheffer DB: Understanding techniques for measuring cardiac output, Biomed Instrum Technol 24:188-197, 1990.
7. American College of Cardiology/American Heart Association Task Force on Assessment of Diagnostic & Therapeutic Cardiovascular Procedures: ACC/AHA guidelines for the clinical application of echocardiography, J Am Coll Clin Cardiol 16.1505-1528, 1990.
8. Drew BJ: Bedside electrocardiographic monitoring: state of the art for the 1990's, Heart Lung 20:610-623, 1991.
9. Goldschlager N, Sox HC Jr: The diagnostic and prognostic value of the treadmill exercise test in the evaluation of chest pain, in patients with recent myocardial infarction, and in asymptomatic individuals, Am Heart J 116:523-535, 1988.
10. Sue DY, Wasserman K: Impact of integrative cardiopulmonary exercise testing on clinical decision making, Chest 99:981-992, 1991.
11. Kramer EL: Lymphoscintigraphy: radiopharmaceutical selection and methods, Nucl Med Biol 17:57-63, 1990.
12. Weissleder R, Thrall JH: The lymphatic system: diagnostic imaging studies, Radiol 172:315-317, 1989.
13. Gibbons RJ: Rest and exercise radionuclide angiography for diagnosis in chronic ischemic heart disease, Circulation 84(suppl 1):I93-I99, 1991.
14. Bayer MF: Effective laboratory evaluation of thyroid status, Med Clin North Am 75:1-26, 1991.
15. Donald RA: The assessment of pituitary function, Clin Biochem 23:23-30, 1990.
16. Tygstrup N: Assessment of liver function: principles and practice, J Gastroenterol Hepatol 5:468-482, 1990.
17. Sallie R, Tredger JM, Williams R: Drugs and the liver. Part 1: testing liver function, Bio Pharm Drug Dispos 12:251-259, 1991.
18. Maglinte DDT, Torres WE, Laufer I: Oral cholecystography in contemporary gallstone imaging: a review, Radiol 178:49-58, 1991.
19. Romano TJ, Dobbins JW: Evaluation of the patient with suspected malabsorption, Gastroenterol Clin North Am 18:467-483, 1989.
20. Quigley EMM: Intestinal manometry: technical advances, clinical limitations, Dig Dis Sci 37:10-13, 1992.
21. Carsons S: Newer laboratory parameters for the diagnosis of rheumatic disease, Am J Med 85(suppl 4A):34-38, 1988.
22. Mackenzie AH: Differential diagnosis of rheumatoid arthritis, Am J Med 85(suppl 4A):2-11, 1988.
23. Silverman GJ, Chen PP, Carson DA: Cold agglutinins: specificity, idiotopy and structural analysis, Chem Immunol 48:109-125, 1990.
24. Atkinson JP: Complement deficiency, Am J Med 85(suppl 6):45-47, 1988.
25. Guerin B, Watson RD: Skin tests, Clin Rev Allergy 6:211-227, 1988.
26. Weinstein AJ, Farkas S: Serologic tests in infectious disease, Med Clin North Am 62:1099-1117, 1978.
27. Habicht J-P, Pelletier DL: The importance of context in choosing nutritional indicators, J Nutr 120:1519-1524, 1990.
28. Sauberlich HE: Implications of nutritional status on human biochemistry, physiology, and health, Clin Biochem 17:132-142, 1984.
29. Starker PM: Nutritional assessment of the hospitalized patient, Adv Nutr Res 8:109-118, 1990.
30. Clark JS et al: Noninvasive assessment of blood gases, Am Rev Respir Dis 145:220-232, 1992.

31. Cushner HM, Copley JB: Review: back to basics: the urinalysis: a selected national survey and review, *Am J Med Sci* 297:193-196, 1989.
32. Haber MH: Quality assurance in urinalysis, *Clin Lab Med* 8:431-447, 1988.
33. Hattery RR et al: Intravenous urographic technique, *Radiol* 167:593-599, 1988.
34. Shure D: Transbronchial biopsy and needle aspiration, *Chest* 95:1130-1138, 1989.
35. Krone KD, Weiner SA: Interpreting chest films, *Hosp Med* 22:205-207, 210, 215-218, 220-222, 225-227, 231, 1987.
36. McCarty DJ: Crystal identification in human synovial fluids, *Rheum Dis Clin North Am* 14:253-267, 1988.

The Patient Case Presentation

6

CHAPTER

- List each component of the patient case presentation.
- State the appropriate sequence for presenting the patient case presentation.
- Given specific patient information, identify its appropriate location in the patient case presentation.
- Identify the appropriate sequence for presenting laboratory and diagnostic test results.

*P*atient information, including the history, physical examination, medication history, laboratory reports, and progress reports, is available from a variety of documented sources (e.g., patient chart) and undocumented sources (e.g., colleagues, patients). Effective written or verbal communication of this sometimes complex patient-specific information is not possible without a universally accepted structure. The structured patient case presentation is the accepted tool for presenting and documenting patient information (Figure 6-1). Primary care providers use the structured patient case format to communicate essential patient information to colleagues and consultants. The structured patient case presentation also is an important teaching tool for students and other trainees who are expected to locate, organize, and present patient-specific information to preceptors or other clinicians. The student or trainee learns to organize and present the patient information, and the preceptor uses the details of the case (as presented) to assess the student's or trainee's understanding of the case.

COMPONENTS

The patient case presentation is an organized summary of all known patient information. Considered an up-to-date "snapshot" of the patient, the patient case presentation provides a thorough and detailed picture of the patient at the time of the presentation (Box 6-1).[1-3] The patient case presentation summarizes important information. A good patient case presentation provides all the information needed to understand the patient case but spares the listener or reader from a barrage of duplicate, trivial, or irrelevant information. The person presenting or writing the patient case identifies and selects the pertinent details and salient information. It takes practice to create thorough, well-organized, smooth-flowing patient case presentations.

General Information and Chief Complaint: CW is a 28-year-old white female who presented to her local medical doctor on 10/21/02 with a chief complaint of "I have a rash."

History of Present Illness: CW complains of an itchy rash that started yesterday. She first noticed the rash on her chest and stomach yesterday morning; the rash spread to her arms and legs last night. The itching kept her awake all night. She felt warm but did not take her temperature. She started taking co-trimoxazole (Bactrim) 2 days ago for a urinary tract infection. She is not taking any other medication and has not used any new soaps, detergents, perfumes, or cosmetics.

Past Medical History: CW is status post a fractured left tibia at the age of 7 years and an appendectomy at the age of 12 years.

Family History: CW's mother is alive and well at the age of 49 years. Her father is alive and well at the age of 51 years; he was recently diagnosed with hypertension. She has three brothers aged 26, 24, and 17 years; all are alive and well.

Social History: CW smokes half a pack of cigarettes daily. She started smoking when she was 21 years of age (7 pack-year history). She drinks three to four beers every weekend and has done so for the past 10 years. She denies the use of recreational or illicit drugs. She is an elementary school teacher and lives by herself in an apartment.

Medication History: CW has no known drug allergies or adverse drug reactions. She started taking Bactrim DS one tablet twice daily on 10/19/02 for a presumed urinary tract infection. Her first dose was at 10 PM on 10/19/02. She took one tablet in the morning and one in the evening on 10/20/02 but did not take this morning's dose. CW uses no other medications routinely and cannot remember the last time she took a prescription drug. She has never taken an herbal product or alternative remedy.

Review of Systems: As per the HPI.

Physical Examination: CW is a pleasant, well-developed, well-nourished WF in no obvious distress. Her vital signs include a blood pressure of 128/72 mm Hg, a heart rate of 88 beats per minute, and a respiratory rate of 10 breaths per minute. Her oral temperature is 99.2 °F. She is 5′ 4″ tall and weighs 52 kg. She has a diffuse maculopapular rash on her trunk and extremities. The lesions are red and flat and range in size from a few millimeters to several large confluent areas (1.5 by 2 cm) on her abdomen and back. The rest of the examination is within normal limits.

Labs: The panel-7 is sodium 140 mEq/L, chloride 108 mEq/L, potassium 4.2 mEq/l, carbon dioxide content 26 mEq/L, blood urea nitrogen 10 mg/dl, and serum creatinine 1.1 mg/dl. The CBC is hemoglobin 14 g/dl, hematocrit 45%, white blood cell count 8500 cells/mm^3 with 53% polymorphonuclear cells, 5% bands, 27% lymphocytes, and 15% eosinophils. The platelets are adequate. The AST is 34 U/L, the ALT is 29 U/L, the alkaline phosphatase is 45U/L, the LDH is 240 U/L, the GGT is 16 U/L, the total bilirubin is 0.8 mg/dl, and the albumin is 5.2 g/dl. Urinalysis from 10/19/02 showed greater than 10^6 organisms per ml; the culture was positive for *E. coli*.

Problem List and Initial Plans
Problem #1—Maculopapular urticarial rash; probably drug related. Discontinue the Bactrim DS and avoid sulfonamide-containing medications. Treat with cool water compresses and lukewarm water baths. Consider an oral antihistamine if the itching persists. Consider a short course of oral corticosteroids if the rash does not resolve.
Problem #2—*E. coli* urinary tract infection. Begin amoxicillin 250 mg every 8 hours for 7 days. Alternatives include amoxicillin-clavulanic acid, cephalosporins, and quinolones. Reculture if still symptomatic at the end of therapy.

Figure 6-1   *Continued*
Example of a Patient Case Presentation.
The patient case presentation is a verbal summary of patient information.

Problem #3—Tobacco smoker. Counsel regarding consequences of smoking and smoking cessation options.
Problem #4—S/P fractured left tibia. Inactive problem.
Problem #5—S/P appendectomy. Inactive problem.

Figure 6-1 cont'd

BOX **6-1**

Sequence and Components of the Patient Case Presentation

1. General information at the time of admission or first contact
   a. Name, age, race, gender
   b. Date of admission or first contact
2. Chief complaint
3. History of present illness
4. Past medical history
5. Family history
6. Social history
7. Medication history
8. Review of systems
9. Physical examination
   a. General descriptive statement
   b. Vital signs
      1. Blood pressure
      2. Heart rate
      3. Temperature
      4. Respiratory rate
   c. Pertinent positive and negative findings on physical examination
10. Pertinent positive and negative laboratory and diagnostic test results
    a. Serum electrolytes (sodium, chloride, carbon dioxide content), creatinine (Cr), blood urea nitrogen (BUN), blood sugar (BS)
    b. Complete blood count (CBC), including white blood cell (WBC) count, differential, hemoglobin (Hgb), hematocrit (HCT), and platelets (PLTS)
    c. Liver function tests (LFTs)
    d. Urinalysis (UA)
    e. Chest x-ray (CXR) film
    f. Electrocardiogram (ECG)
    g. Other test results
11. Patient problem list and initial plans
12. Patient progress
13. Discharge data (if applicable)
    a. Final diagnosis
    b. Discharge medications
14. Plans for follow-up

By convention, each component of the patient case presentation is identified by an abbreviation (Table 6-1). These abbreviations not only are used to document the patient case information in the medical record but also are sometimes used during the case presentation. For example, the person presenting the patient case may say "C-C" instead of "chief complaint," "H-P-I" instead of "history of present illness," and "P-M-H" instead of "past medical history."

The sequence of presentation is standardized (Box 6-2). The sequence is designed to provide a logical flow of information, starting with information about the current medical issue and finishing with an update on the patient's progress. Listeners and readers relax and listen to or read the information presented when they recognize that the information is presented in the standardized format. Details may be overlooked if the listener or reader has to piece the patient information together or worry about missing important details of the case.

GENERAL PATIENT INFORMATION

General patient information includes the date and time of admission to the hospital or arrival at the clinic or office and the patient's name, age, race, and gender.

CHIEF COMPLAINT

The chief complaint (CC) is the reason the patient is seeking medical care. It is presented and documented in the patient's own words, which provides a sense of the patient's experiences and understanding of the problem and conveys the patient's perception of the urgency and severity of the problem. The patient's own words also provide important information regarding level of education and medical sophistication. For example, few patients have a chief complaint of "I think I am having a myocardial infarction." Patients are more likely to complain of heavy, squeezing, or crushing chest pain and discomfort. However, patients with chronic disease and/or repeated contact with the health care system and patients who are health care professionals may use sophisticated medical terminology. A patient who has personally experienced a myocardial infarction or a health care professional might present to the emergency room with the "I think I am having a myocardial infarction" chief complaint.

The chief complaint does not come from comatose or otherwise nonverbal patients. The patient's family or friends may be able to describe the patient's problem; this information is sometimes presented as the chief complaint with a notation of the person supplying the information (e.g., "The patient's wife found him unconscious on the living room floor"). Patients referred for specific tests, procedures, and evaluations

---

TABLE 6-1

Patient Case Abbreviations

Abbreviation	Meaning	Abbreviation	Meaning
CC	Chief complaint	ROS	Review of systems
HPI	History of present illness	MedHx	Medication history
PMH	Past medical history	PE	Physical examination
FH	Family history	Labs	Laboratory and
SH	Social history		diagnostic test results

BOX **6-2**

Suggested Sequence for Presentation of Information during the Patient Case Presentation

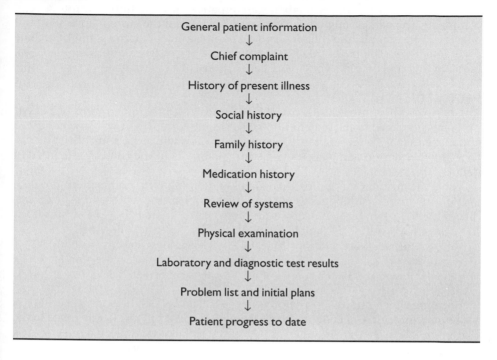

General patient information
↓
Chief complaint
↓
History of present illness
↓
Social history
↓
Family history
↓
Medication history
↓
Review of systems
↓
Physical examination
↓
Laboratory and diagnostic test results
↓
Problem list and initial plans
↓
Patient progress to date

may not offer a chief complaint. If this is the case, the chief complaint is presented as "Referred for _____" (e.g., "referred for cardiac catheterization").

HISTORY OF PRESENT ILLNESS

The history of present illness (HPI) is a narrative that describes the story of the current problem. All characteristic details, such as the specific symptoms, how the problem began or was first recognized, the duration of symptoms, test results from previous evaluations for the same problem, activities and treatments that ease and worsen the problem, and past experiences with the problem, are included in the HPI. Pertinent data from previous hospitalizations and interventions for the same problem, such as dates of admission and discharge, results of tests and diagnostic procedures, medications used to treat the problem, and physiologic data such as serum creatinine and arterial blood gases, are summarized in the HPI.

The HPI is presented in a logical and temporally appropriate sequence. Enough detail is presented to describe the problem, but excessive and repetitive detail is avoided. For example, information presented about pain includes the location, onset, quality (sharp, dull), severity (mild, moderate, severe), duration (acute, chronic), where the pain radiates, and interventions that ease and worsen the pain (e.g., elevation, warmth, cold, food, water, medications).

Risk factors for diseases and conditions such as myocardial infarction, hypertension, diabetes mellitus, and tuberculosis are included in the HPI if the patient has been diagnosed with one of these diseases or if the chief complaint suggests a problem with known risk factors. For example, information regarding a family history of cardiac disease and the patient's history of hypertension, smoking, and previous myocardial infarctions is presented if myocardial infarction is suspected.

The HPI also includes pertinent negative patient information—symptoms and complaints the patient might be expected to have given the current complaint but does not. For example, the HPI for a patient complaining of dizziness might include a statement that the patient does not have a history of fever, vomiting, diarrhea, blood in the stool or urine, chest pain, palpitations, or head trauma.

PAST MEDICAL HISTORY

The past (or prior) medical history (PMH) includes a brief description of patient problems unrelated to the present illness. For example, a patient with hypertension and diabetes may be seeking care for complaints of cough, fever, and chills. The history of hypertension and diabetes is mentioned briefly in the HPI but presented in detail in the PMH.

The PMH includes the approximate dates and duration for each patient problem and information regarding surgical and other major medical procedures (e.g., cardiac catheterization, bronchoscopy, skin biopsy). The abbreviation *S/P* (status post) indicates a past event. For example, the PMH may include the following:

Mild to moderate hypertension for 10 years; insulin-dependent diabetes mellitus for 5 years; glaucoma for 25 years; S/P fractured left tibia in 1979; S/P three-vessel CABG [coronary artery bypass graft] in November 1985; S/P T&A [tonsillectomy and adenoidectomy] as a child.

Deciding which information belongs in the HPI and which belongs in the PMH is sometimes difficult. Generally, if details from the patient's PMH directly relate to the current problem, they are included as part of the HPI. For example, if a patient has a chief complaint of angina, details from the patient's history regarding previous myocardial infarctions and cardiac bypass surgery are included in the HPI in addition to being mentioned in the PMH.

SOCIAL HISTORY

The social history (SH) contains information about the patient's use of tobacco, alcohol, and illicit drugs. It also contains information about the patient's occupation, marital status, sexual history, and living conditions.

Tobacco use is quantified in packs per day and pack-years. (Refer to Chapter 3 for information regarding how to express a patient's smoking history in pack-years.) The approximate start and stop dates, as well as the reason for stopping, are noted for tobacco, alcohol, and each illicit drug.

The type, amount, pattern, and duration of alcohol ingestion are described in the SH. For example, alcohol consumption may be described as "a fifth of whiskey daily for the past 15 years" or "a case of beer every weekend for 6 years." The term *social drinking* is sometimes used to describe the drinking habits of patients who do not drink regularly but only if dining out and attending other social occasions. However, the term *social drinking* is open to wide interpretation. The person presenting the case should quantify the type, amount, pattern, and duration of alcohol ingestion. The date and time of the last drink is noted for patients who drink regularly.

The use of illicit, or so-called recreational or street, drugs may be documented in the SH instead of or in place of documenting this information in the medication history. As with the documentation of alcohol use, the amount, pattern, and duration of use of these agents are described in the SH. For example, "The patient smokes marijuana every weekend and has done so for 8 years" or "The patient uses crack cocaine daily and has done so for 3 years." As with documentation of tobacco, the date of the last use of these drugs is presented (e.g., "The patient last used cocaine this morning").

The patient's occupation is documented in the SH. This information is important for both diagnostic reasoning and therapeutic planning. For example, a 40-year history of working in a naval shipyard may be an important piece of information for a patient with pulmonary complaints consistent with mesothelioma. Knowing a patient's work schedule and environment before making decisions regarding the best therapeutic regimen for the patient also may be helpful. For example, the selection of a diuretic as the initial drug treatment for a patient with mild to moderate hypertension may not be the best choice if the patient has a work schedule that precludes frequent rest room breaks. Some jobs, such as assembly line factory jobs, do not permit much individual privacy; patients with these types of jobs may be reluctant to be seen taking medication. Compliance for these patients may be enhanced by selecting medications with dosing schedules that permit the medication to be taken in the privacy of the home.

The patient's living conditions are documented in the SH. For example, the person presenting the case may note that the patient lives at home with a spouse and children or is currently living in a homeless shelter. For patients with physically limiting diseases such as rheumatoid arthritis and emphysema, information regarding the layout of the house is an important part of the SH.

FAMILY HISTORY

The family history (FH) consists of a brief summary of the medical histories of the patient's first-degree relatives (parents, siblings, and offspring). Data presented in the FH include information regarding the status (alive or dead) of the patient's parents, siblings, and children; cause of death and age at death for family members who have died; and current health problems of living family members.

A number of abbreviations and shorthand notations are used for the FH. These abbreviations are not verbally presented but are used to document the FH in the written medical record. Common abbreviations include M for mother, F for father, B for brother, and S for sister. An arrow pointing up ($\uparrow$) indicates the individual is alive; an arrow pointing down ($\downarrow$) indicates the individual is dead. For example, the notation *M$\downarrow$78(MI)* indicates the patient's mother died at the age of 78 from a myocardial infarction.

The FH may be detailed and well documented for several generations if the patient is suspected of having a genetically linked disease. The patient's family pedigree is documented by using a set of universally recognized symbols (Figure 6-2). The age of each relative may be noted near the symbol.

MEDICATION HISTORY

Most medication histories obtained and documented by nonpharmacist health care professionals lack the detail of those obtained and documented by pharmacists. Therefore the pharmacist should include the detailed information obtained from the patient medication history interview when making patient case presentations. (See Chapter 3 for information regarding the patient medication history and Box 3-4 for specific data included in the medication history.)

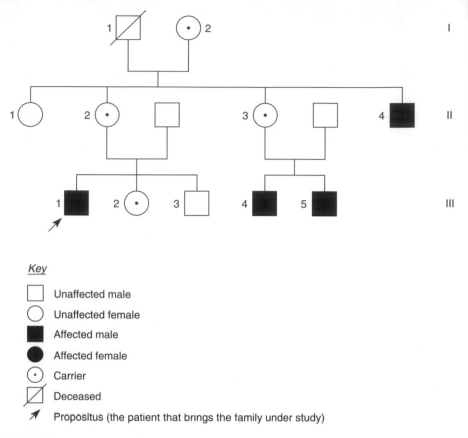

Figure 6-2
Family Pedigrees.
Family pedigrees provide information about genetically linked diseases and their transmission across generations. Roman numerals indicate generation. Arabic numerals provide patient reference numbers within each generation.

REVIEW OF SYSTEMS

The review of systems (ROS) summarizes all current patient complaints not included in the HPI. It typically follows an organ system approach (e.g., head, heart, lung); pertinent positive findings are presented. For example, a patient may have a chief complaint of cough and fever but, when asked about other complaints or problems, may identify chronic constipation. In this example the story of the cough and fever is described in the HPI and the story of the chronic constipation is described in the ROS.

PHYSICAL EXAMINATION

Presentation of the physical examination (PE) typically begins with a short description of the patient. The patient description helps listeners or readers visualize the patient and begin to anticipate pertinent findings. The listener or reader formulates different impressions and anticipates the presentation of substantially different data from the PE based on the initial patient description. Note the difference in the impressions given by the following descriptions of patients A and B:

Patient A is a pleasant, cooperative 48-year-old African-American female in mild respiratory distress. Patient B is a white female of unknown age who is unconscious and intubated.

The patient's vital signs, including the blood pressure and heart rate (supine, sitting, or standing as indicated by the patient's initial complaint), respiratory rate, and temperature follow the initial description of the patient.

Pertinent positive and negative findings from the PE are presented next (see Chapter 4 for information regarding physical assessment). Pertinent positive findings such as abnormalities found on PE and pertinent negative findings such as abnormalities expected to have been found on PE given the patient's complaints or current or potential medical problems that were absent on examination are presented in an organized sequence and format. For example, a logical sequence of presentation of this information is to present the findings from the skin; head, eyes, ears, nose, and throat (HEENT); heart; chest; abdomen; genitalia; and extremities. Findings from the neurologic examination are presented last.

LABORATORY AND DIAGNOSTIC TEST RESULTS

Results from laboratory and diagnostic tests and procedures are presented after the physical assessment section of the patient case (see Chapter 5 for information regarding laboratory and diagnostic tests and procedures). The amount of detail included in the laboratory and diagnostic test result section depends on the severity and complexity of the patient's medical problem. In some simple, straightforward patient cases, simply stating that all laboratory findings or all laboratory findings except one specific test, such as the chest x-ray film, were within normal limits may be sufficient. However, many clinicians want to know all baseline laboratory patient data. Students and trainees may be expected to present and comment on every laboratory and diagnostic test and procedure reported for the patient.

There is no single universally accepted sequence for presenting laboratory and diagnostic test results. However, common laboratory test results typically are presented first. For example, a common sequence is to present the serum electrolytes (sodium, chloride, potassium, carbon dioxide content), glucose, blood urea nitrogen, and creatinine first (panel-7, SMA-6), followed by the complete cell count (white blood cells with differential, hemoglobin, hematocrit, platelets), other electrolytes and serum chemistries, and macroscopic and microscopic urinalysis. Nonroutine laboratory test results are presented next, followed by a description of electrocardiograms, radiographs, and other diagnostic tests and procedures.

PATIENT PROBLEM LIST

The patient problem list and initial diagnostic and therapeutic plans are presented after the presentation of laboratory and diagnostic test results. The patient problem list is a brief listing of the patient's problems, starting with the most acute problem (see Chapter 7 for information regarding problem identification, prioritization, therapeutic planning, and monitoring). It is not uncommon for different health care professionals to come up with different patient problem lists for the same patient case. For example, pharmacists often include patient nonadherence, chronic health evaluation issues (e.g., routine immunizations, monthly breast self-exams, blood pressure screening), and chronic anticoagulation on the patient problem list.

PROGRESS

All the information presented so far describes the initial case presentation presented at the time of first contact with the patient. However, a great deal more information is available for patients who have been hospitalized or for patients who have had numerous office or clinic visits for the same medical problem. A patient case presentation may be made at any point in the care of the patient. Information obtained after the initial patient admission or clinic visit presentation is presented at the end of the patient case presentation in a logical, temporal sequence. The patient case presentation for a hospitalized patient includes the initial patient case information plus a summary of data obtained during the current hospitalization. For example, presenting every vital sign documented for a patient who has been hospitalized for several days for the management of hypertension is tedious and unnecessary. These data are summarized for the case presentation so that trends and links between treatment and outcomes are identified.

OTHER INFORMATION

Additional information beyond that described in this chapter is presented as part of the patient case presentation when applicable. This information, which may include plans for additional diagnostic procedures and therapeutic interventions, discharge plans, plans for follow-up after discharge from the hospital, and autopsy results, is presented at the end of the patient case presentation.

SELF-ASSESSMENT QUESTIONS

1. A patient had an appendectomy 40 years ago. This information belongs in which section of the patient case?
    a. HPI
    b. PMH
    c. SH
    d. FH
    e. ROS
2. Which of the following is presented first when presenting the physical assessment section of the patient case?
    a. General descriptive statement
    b. Neurologic
    c. Cardiovascular
    d. HEENT
    e. Pulmonary
3. A patient goes to the local medical doctor with angina. The patient states having several migraine headaches per year. The information about the migraine headaches belongs in which section of the patient case?
    a. HPI
    b. SH
    c. FH
    d. ROS
    e. Laboratory and diagnostic test results
4. Vital signs include all of the following except:
    a. Blood pressure
    b. Cardiac output
    c. Temperature
    d. Respiratory rate
    e. Heart rate

5. A patient's 96-year-old mother is alive and well. This information belongs in which section of the patient case?
    a. HPI
    b. PMH
    c. SH
    d. FH
    e. ROS

6. Which of the following laboratory test results should be presented first in the patient case presentation?
    a. Chest x-ray film
    b. Urinalysis
    c. Serum electrolytes
    d. Electrocardiogram
    e. Hemoglobin

7. Which of the following is presented first in the patient case presentation?
    a. Patient progress
    b. CC
    c. PE
    d. HPI
    e. Medication history

8. Which of the following is presented last in the patient case presentation?
    a. Patient progress
    b. CC
    c. PE
    d. HPI
    e. Medication history

9. In a family pedigree, what does a closed box with a slash indicate?
    a. Unaffected living male
    b. Affected living male
    c. Unaffected deceased male
    d. Affected deceased male
    e. Propositus

10. A 42-year-old man is admitted with a suspected myocardial infarction. His risk factors for myocardial infarction (smoking, hypertension, positive family history, hypercholesterolemia, and obesity) are listed in which section of the patient case presentation?
    a. HPI
    b. PMH
    c. SH
    d. FH
    e. ROS

References

1. Kassirer JP, Kopelman RI: The case presentation: 1. Principles, Hosp Pract 23:21, 25-26, 29, 1988.
2. Kihm JT et al: Quantitative analysis of the outpatient oral case presentation, J Gen Intern Med 6:233-236, 1991.
3. Yurchak PM: A guide to medical case presentations, Res Staff Phys 27:109-111, 114-115, 1981.

Therapeutics Planning

7

CHAPTER

Learning Objectives

- List the planning process components.
- List the steps involved in patient problem identification.
- Identify subjective and objective patient parameters.
- List the steps involved in problem prioritization.
- Prioritize patient problems.
- List the steps involved in the selection of specific therapeutic regimens.
- Select patient-specific therapeutic regimens.
- Describe the subjective, objective, assessment, and plan (SOAP) format.

*P*lanning is the heart of the decision-making process. Effective planning facilitates the selection of appropriate medication regimens for specific patient problems and provides a framework for monitoring a patient's response to therapy.

The planning process consists of problem identification and prioritization, selection of treatment regimens for each patient problem, and development of an integrated monitoring plan (Box 7-1). Planning also incorporates well-thought-out alternative treatment regimens. Successful planning requires expert knowledge of pharmacotherapeutics, human disease, physical assessment, and laboratory and diagnostic tests (Figure 7-1). Planning incorporates consideration of patient factors that influence therapeutic regimens (e.g., history of nonadherence to medication regimens) as well as consideration of how medications influence patients (e.g., drowsiness). This chapter describes problem identification and prioritization and selection of specific medication regimens; monitoring is discussed in Chapter 8.

PROBLEM IDENTIFICATION

Consider all available data from the patient's history, physical examination, laboratory and diagnostic tests, and the pharmacist-acquired medication history when identifying patient problems. Group related subjective and objective parameters to determine specific patient problems.

BOX 7-1

The Planning Process

1. Problem identification
   Step 1—Identify subjective and objective patient parameters.
   Step 2—Group related parameters.
   Step 3—Assess the parameters and determine the specific patient problems.
2. Problem prioritization
   Step 1—Identify the active problems.
   Step 2—Identify the inactive problems.
   Step 3—Rank the problems.
3. Selection of specific therapeutic regimens
   Step 1—Create a list of therapeutic options.
   Step 2—Eliminate drugs from the list based on patient-specific and external factors.
   Step 3—Select dosage, route, and duration of therapy.
   Step 4—Identify alternative therapeutic regimens.
4. Monitoring
   Step 1—Set therapeutic goals.
   Step 2—Determine patient- and drug-specific monitoring parameters.
   Step 3—Integrate the monitoring plan.
   Step 4—Obtain data.
   Step 5—Assess the response to therapy.

STEP 1—IDENTIFY PATIENT PARAMETERS FROM THE MEDICAL HISTORY, PHYSICAL EXAMINATION, LABORATORY AND DIAGNOSTIC TESTS, AND THE PHARMACIST-ACQUIRED MEDICATION HISTORY

Create a working list of all available subjective and objective data. Identifying relevant subjective and objective parameters from the medication history, history of present illness, past medical history, social history, review of systems, physical examination, and laboratory and diagnostic tests requires patience and methodical scrutiny. It is important to consider all available data. Patient factors that by themselves appear unimportant may be important when considered in the context of other patient data. *Pertinent positive* data, including abnormalities such as a serum potassium that exceeds the upper limit of the reference range (e.g., serum potassium of 5.8 mEq/L) or a patient's description of signs and symptoms of a migraine headache, are relatively easy to identify. *Pertinent negative* data, that is, objective or subjective data that are normal but would be expected to be abnormal given the patient's disease or condition, are more difficult to recognize and require a good understanding of human disease and pharmacotherapeutics. For example, many patients with long-standing type 1 diabetes mellitus have diabetic retinopathy. The fact that a patient with long-standing type 1 diabetes mellitus does not have diabetic retinopathy is important pertinent negative data.

Subjective parameters, such as coughing, pain, and itching, are describable but cannot be precisely measured or quantified (Box 7-2). *Objective parameters*, such as blood pressure, heart rate, and temperature, can be precisely measured or quantified (Box 7-3). Subjective parameters may be less obvious and more difficult to identify. Conventionally, parameters such as crackles, edema, and muscle atrophy that are

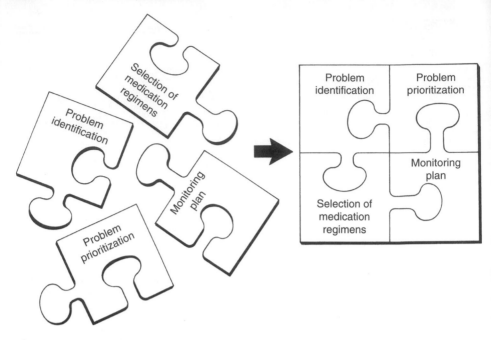

Figure 7-1
Components of Therapeutics Planning.
Therapeutics planning consists of problem identification and prioritization, selection of specific initial and alternative medication regimens for patient problems, and development of a monitoring plan.

observed by the health care professional during the physical examination but cannot be precisely quantified are considered objective parameters.

STEP 2—CREATE SETS OF RELATED PARAMETERS
Evaluate the list of objective and subjective parameters for possible relationships among the parameters. Identify related abnormalities that combine to indicate specific patient problems. For example, subjective complaints of fever, one episode of chills, and productive cough combined with objective data of leukocytosis with an increased percentage of bands, a chest x-ray film showing right middle lobe consolidation, and sputum positive for gram-positive encapsulated cocci in pairs are related.

STEP 3—DETERMINE SPECIFIC PATIENT PROBLEMS
Evaluate each group of related subjective and objective parameters to determine the specific patient problem or issue. Patient problems include current medical problems such as hypertension, pneumonia, asthma, diabetes, and gastrointestinal bleeding; past medical problems such as a history of migraine headache, hip fracture, deep vein thrombosis, and myocardial infarction; past surgeries such as appendectomy, tonsillectomy, coronary artery bypass grafts, and transurethral resection of the prostate; and issues such as noncompliance, obesity, drug abuse, and allergies. Some pharmacists consider corticosteroid dependency and chronic anticoagulation therapy

BOX **7-2**

Common Subjective Parameters

Anxiety	Headache	Palpitations
Bloating	Heartburn	Pounding pulse
Blood-tinged sputum	Heat intolerance	Rash
Blurred vision	Impotence	Seizures
Breast tenderness	Indigestion	Shortness of breath
Chills	Insomnia	Slurred speech
Cold intolerance	Incontinence	Sneezing
Confusion	Itching	Sore throat
Constipation	Joint pain	Syncope
Cramps	Loss of appetite	Thirst
Decreased appetite	Loss of libido	Tingling
Depression	Muscle aches	Tinnitus
Diarrhea	Muscle weakness	Tremor
Difficulty concentrating	Nasal congestion	Vertigo
Dry skin	Nasal itching	Weakness
Dysuria	Nausea	Wheezing
Fatigue	Nervousness	
Flatulence	Numbness	

BOX **7-3**

Common Objective Parameters

Height and weight

Vital signs—temperature, blood pressure, heart rate, respiratory rate

Blood chemistries—sodium, potassium, chloride, carbon dioxide content, glucose, creatinine, aspartate aminotransferase, alanine aminotransferase, bilirubin, calcium, magnesium, cholesterol, triglycerides, alkaline phosphatase, lactic dehydrogenase, uric acid, urea nitrogen

Blood gases—pH, P_{CO_2}, P_{O_2}, bicarbonate

Blood proteins—total protein, albumin, complements, immunoglobulins

Hematology—hemoglobin, hematocrit, mean corpuscular volume, mean corpuscular hemoglobin concentration, red blood cell count, white blood cell count and differential

Urinalysis—specific gravity, cellular content, protein

Cultures and sensitivities—blood, urine, sputum, tissue

Serum drug concentrations

Specific organ system tests—peak expiratory flow rate, forced expiratory volume in 1 second and forced vital capacity (and the ratio of the two), ejection fraction, triiodothyronine, thyroxine, thyroid-stimulating hormone, creatinine clearance

Miscellaneous—urine output, abdominal girth, number of loose stools per day, input and output

identifiable problems and separate them from the medical problems that prompted the drug therapy such as steroid-dependent asthma and recurrent thrombophlebitis. In the example in step 3, the data suggests a bacterial pneumonia, most likely *Streptococcus pneumoniae*.

PROBLEM PRIORITIZATION

The second step in the planning process is prioritization of the patient problems. Prioritization means ranking patient problems with the most urgent problems on the top of the list and the least urgent problems on the bottom. Prioritization is a way of ordering the relative acuteness of the problems and is not meant to imply a rank ordering of importance or significance to the patient's overall health care needs.

STEP 1—IDENTIFY THE ACTIVE PROBLEMS
Active problems require some kind of drug or nondrug intervention. Examples of active problems include pneumonia, asthma, congestive heart failure, trauma, cerebrovascular accident, myocardial infarction, and anxiety.

STEP 2—IDENTIFY THE INACTIVE PROBLEMS
Inactive problems are of historical interest only and do not require drug or nondrug intervention. Examples of inactive problems include a history of an appendectomy at age 12, a history of pneumonia 2 years ago, a history of smoking two packs of cigarettes per day until quitting 10 years ago, and a history of sulfa-associated rash. Although inactive problems do not require planning for drug or nondrug therapy, inactive problems need to be identified and listed so that they can be considered when planning for treatment of active problems. For example, a patient with a history of splenectomy is at increased risk of infections with *Streptococcus pneumoniae*, *Haemophilus influenzae*, *Neisseria meningitidis*, and some gram-negative bacteria. Knowledge of this risk will help in planning patient-specific antibiotic therapy in the event the patient presents with signs and symptoms consistent with infection.

STEP 3—RANK THE PROBLEMS
One approach to ranking patient problems is to identify the problem that needs the most immediate attention and then rank the remaining problems in order of need for intervention. The number one problem is the problem that if left untreated will cause the most harm to the patient in the shortest amount of time. For example, consider a patient with bacterial meningitis, obesity, and a history of a broken leg as a child. The bacterial meningitis is clearly the most acute life-threatening problem. The obesity is active but not as immediately life-threatening as the meningitis. The history of a broken leg as a child is an inactive problem and is ranked at the bottom of the list. Another approach is to work from the bottom of the list, determining the problem requiring the least attention. This problem is ranked as the least important problem. The pharmacist repeats the ranking process with the remaining problems until all are ranked. Regardless of the approach used, the active problems are at the top of the list, inactive problems are at the bottom, and active but less acute problems are in the middle. The rank ordering is a rather arbitrary process if the problems all have relatively equal acuity.

Pharmacists given the same list of patient problems may develop different prioritized lists. This is not unexpected; no one list is correct. Lists are developed based on the clinical judgment and experience of the practitioner. In addition, because the focus of the pharmacist is on therapeutic issues rather than on differential diagnosis, the pharmacist-generated patient problem list may be similar although not necessarily identical to the problem list generated by physicians, nurses, or other health care professionals.

SELECTION OF SPECIFIC THERAPEUTIC REGIMENS

Select specific therapeutic regimens for each patient problem, including initial and alternative medication regimens, after the patient problems are identified and prioritized. Determine the most appropriate medication or combination of medications for the management of each problem. The recommendation includes the specific medication, dosage, route of administration, dosage formulation, duration of therapy, and rationale. The general approach is to develop the therapeutic plan for each problem and then integrate the individual plans, making sure that each component of the integrated plan is achievable for the specific patient.

Selection of a specific regimen requires assessment of each patient problem in the context of information known about the patient as well as external factors. Consider interventions that have and have not worked for the patient in the past, the influence of other patient problems on the proposed medication regimen, and the influence of the proposed regimen on all other patient problems (Box 7-4). For example, a patient who has responded well to a specific decongestant in the past will most likely respond well to the same decongestant in the future. A patient with renal insufficiency is at risk of developing seizures from the accumulation of normeperidine, a renally eliminated metabolite of meperidine. A drug with negative inotropic effects may worsen a patient's congestive heart failure.

Consider external factors, including the current state-of-the-art therapeutics for managing the specific problem, cost considerations, and limitations imposed by institutional and state formularies, when selecting an optimal therapeutic regimen. Rarely is any single therapeutic regimen the only possible appropriate regimen; many different regimens may be equally effective for the patient. The decision between equally effective regimens is based on experience, personal preference, and consideration of external limitations such as restrictive drug formularies or cost.

STEP 1—CREATE A LIST OF THERAPEUTIC OPTIONS FOR EACH PROBLEM

Identify all classes of drugs and possible therapeutic approaches for each problem; do not eliminate any option at this stage of planning. This step may require review of current pharmacotherapeutics and human disease textbooks, literature searches of the current pharmacy and medical literature, or consultation with colleagues. This step becomes easier and more time efficient with practice and experience.

STEP 2—ELIMINATE THERAPEUTIC OPTIONS FROM THE LIST CREATED IN STEP 1

Once all therapeutic options are identified, eliminate options based on the comparative effectiveness of the drugs; the suitability of the drug for the patient given the other patient problems; the ability of the patient to comply with the proposed regimen; and other factors such as the effectiveness of previous treatment regimens, cost, and formulary restrictions. Consider the impact of the therapeutic option on other patient problems (e.g., the adverse effect of beta-adrenergic blocker antihyper-

BOX 7-4

Factors to Consider When Selecting a Specific Therapeutic Regimen

PATIENT-SPECIFIC FACTORS
What regimens have effectively managed the problem in the past?
What regimens have not effectively managed the problem in the past?
How might other patient problems influence the proposed regimen?
How might the proposed regimen influence other patient problems?

EXTERNAL FACTORS
Current "state-of-the-art" therapeutics
Cost of the proposed therapy
Formulary limitations

tensives on patients with asthma) and the influence of other patient problems on the therapeutic option (e.g., the need to reduce the dosage in a patient with chronic renal insufficiency).

STEP 3—SELECT AN APPROPRIATE THERAPEUTIC REGIMEN FOR EACH PROBLEM
Decisions about the most appropriate medication regimen are based on past patient experiences, assessment of the severity of the problem, drug-specific factors such as the therapeutic index of the drug, and specific patient factors such as chronic renal or hepatic disease that may influence the elimination or metabolism of the drug. Determine the best drug and nondrug regimen, including each specific drug, dose, route, duration of therapy, and rationale for why each drug and nondrug component of the regimen was selected.

STEP 4—IDENTIFY ALTERNATIVE REGIMENS
An important part of the planning process includes anticipation of potential patient problems. A well-constructed plan includes alternative medication regimens for common potential problems, such as the development of an allergy or adverse reaction to the initial therapeutic regimen, lack of desired therapeutic response to the initial therapeutic regimen, and additional patient problems influencing the effectiveness or pharmacokinetics of the initial therapeutic regimen. Anticipation of these potential problems allows for the creation of well-thought-out alternative therapeutic plans instead of therapeutic plans hastily chosen when unanticipated patient problems appear. For example, therapeutic planning for a patient with newly diagnosed hypertension must include plans for alternative therapeutic regimens if the initial treatment fails to lower the blood pressure or must be discontinued because of the development of intolerable side effects.

SOAPING FORMAT
The process of identifying the subjective and objective data, assessing the problem, and developing a specific therapeutic and monitoring plan is called *SOAPing the problem*. The term *SOAP* is an acronym for *s*ubjective, *o*bjective, *a*ssessment, and *p*lan.

The SOAP format provides a formal organizational structure. The steps for SOAPing a problem include the following:

1. Creating a list of related subjective parameters
2. Creating a list of related objective parameters
3. Assessing and documenting the problem
4. Documenting the therapeutic plan for addressing the problem

Commonly, each problem is SOAPed individually, although some clinicians prefer to integrate all data and plans into a single SOAP note.

▪ *Patient Case Example—Integration and Application* ▪

The steps involved in therapeutics planning (problem identification, problem prioritization, and selection of initial and alternative medication regimens) are illustrated in the following patient case.

Patient Case

Date: Late August
Setting: Outpatient Clinic
Chief complaint: "There has to be something you can do for my allergies."
History of present illness: LS is a 31 y/o F with a 20+ year history of seasonal allergic rhinitis (SAR) and type 2 diabetes mellitus. She is allergic to ragweed and has symptoms every fall but claims that this fall is much worse than usual. She complains of multiple bouts of sneezing, runny nose, fatigue, irritability, and itchy eyes, nose, and throat. Her symptoms are worse when she is outside and better when she's inside air-conditioned buildings. She's had to trade out of recess duty at work and has not been able to attend her children's soccer games. She has taken every available prescription antihistamine but feels they are not as effective as the nonprescription antihistamines. However, nonprescription antihistamines make her too drowsy to work or drive, so she doesn't take many doses. She started taking nasal cromolyn QID a couple of weeks ago. She has taken several short courses of oral steroids in the past but hasn't taken any for several years. She tries to avoid steroids because they make her diabetes hard to control. Her last influenza vaccine was 4 years ago. She denies fever, sore throat, cough, vomiting, or diarrhea.
Past medical history: Type 2 diabetes mellitus × 10 years controlled with oral medications and diet.
Social history: Married, four children (sons 8 & 10 and daughters 4 & 5). Lives in a two-story house in the suburbs. No tobacco, no alcohol, no illicit drugs. Elementary school teacher (teaches 1st grade).
Family history: M↑ (50 w/ SAR, asthma), F↑ (51 w/ SAR); two siblings with SAR. All four of her children have SAR.
Review of systems: As per HPI.

Medication History

Dietary: ADA diet.
Allergies: NKDA.
Adverse drug reactions: None.
Current prescription medications:
    Glucophage (metformin) 1000 mg BID × 5 years.

Continued

Past prescription medications:
>   Has tried "every prescription antihistamine available." She says that they "sort of work" but are not as effective as the nonprescription antihistamines.
>   Several different medications for the type 2 DM but cannot remember their names. Has had to use insulin a couple of times while taking prednisone.
>   Prednisone for a few days "when my allergies are really bad"; cannot remember exact dosages or dates.

Current nonprescription medications:
>   Benadryl Allergy (diphenhydramine) 25 mg once or twice a day, mostly in the evenings or at night; started about 2 weeks ago.
>   Nasalcrom (cromolyn sodium) 1 spray each nostril QID during fall allergy season × 2 years; started about 2 weeks ago.

Current and Past Alternative Remedies: No current alternative remedies. Has tried Devil's Claw, pollen extracts, and echinacea for her allergies without noticeable benefit.

Compliance: Takes her medications as prescribed or recommended.

Physical Examination

LS is a pleasant but uncomfortable-appearing woman. She is 5'1" tall and weighs 180 lbs.

Vital Signs: Afebrile; BP 114/74 mm Hg; HR 72 BPM, RR 10 BPM

Head, eyes, ears, nose, and throat: PERRLA, EOMI, TM intact; + conjunctival injection; + chemosis; + rhinorrhea (clear watery secretions); pale, swollen nasal mucosa; oropharynx clear except for some postnasal drip; + periorbital edema; + allergic shiners; + allergic crease

Cardiovascular: RRR; S_1, S_2; PMI5ICS MCL; no murmurs, rubs, or gallops

Lungs: CTA

Abdomen: NABS; NTND

Neurologic system: A&O ×3; cranial nerve II-XII intact

Extremities: Strength 5/5 UE and LE; reflexes 2+ UE and LE

Laboratory Tests and Diagnostic Procedures

Today's labs: Random fingerstick blood glucose 150 mg/dl

Labs from last visit 5 months ago: HbA_{1C} 6%

Problem Identification

Step 1. Identify subjective and objective parameters.

Subjective parameters include the following:

- "There has to be something you can do for my allergies."
- Allergy symptoms are worse than usual
- 20+ year hx of SAR
- Type 2 DM × 10 yrs
- Allergic to ragweed
- Multiple bouts of sneezing
- Runny nose
- Fatigue
- Irritability
- Itchy eyes, nose, and throat
- Allergy symptoms are worse outside
- Traded out of recess duty
- Unable to attend children's soccer games
- Feels better inside air-conditioned buildings

- Has taken all available prescription antihistamines but not as effective as nonprescription antihistamines
- Nonprescription antihistamines make her too drowsy to work or drive so limits use
- Nasal cromolyn QID × 2 wks
- Has taken several courses of oral steroids in past
- Prednisone increases her blood glucose; has had to use insulin in the past
- Last influenza vaccine was 4 yrs ago
- No fevers, sore throat, cough, vomiting, or diarrhea
- Follows the ADA diet
- + FH for SAR (parents, siblings, and children)
- Glucophage 1000 mg BID × 5 yrs
- Prednisone for a few days in past
- Benadryl Allergy 25 mg 1-2×/day for about 2 wks
- Nasalcrom 1 spray each nostril QID for about 2 wks
- Has tried Devil's Claw, pollen extracts, echinacea in the past without noticeable improvement

Objective parameters include the following:

- 5'1"
- 180 lbs.
- + Conjunctival injection
- + Chemosis
- + Rhinorrhea (clear, watery secretions)
- Pale, swollen nasal mucosa
- Oropharynx clear except for postnasal drip
- + Periorbital edema
- + Allergic shiners
- + Allergic crease
- Random fingerstick glucose 150 mg/dl
- HbA_{1C} 6% 5 months ago

Step 2. Group related parameters.

1. Allergy Group

    Subjective parameters: "There has to be something you can do for my allergies"; allergy symptoms are worse than usual; 20+ year hx of SAR; allergic to ragweed; multiple bouts of sneezing; runny nose; fatigue; irritability; itchy eyes, nose, and throat; allergy symptoms are worse outside; traded out of recess duty; unable to attend children's soccer games; feels better inside air-conditioned buildings; has taken all available prescription antihistamines but not as effective as nonprescription antihistamines; nonprescription antihistamines make her too drowsy to work of drive so limits use; nasal cromolyn QID × 2 wks; has taken several courses of oral steroids in past; prednisone increases her blood glucose; has had to use insulin in the past; no fevers, sore throat, cough, vomiting, or diarrhea; + FH for SAR (parents, siblings, and children); prednisone for a few days in past; Benadryl Allergy 25 mg 1-2×/day for about 2 wks; Nasalcrom 1 spray each nostril QID for about 2 wks; has tried Devil's Claw, pollen extracts, echinacea in the past without noticeable improvement.

    Objective parameters: + conjunctival injection; + chemosis; + nasal congestion; + rhinorrhea (clear, watery secretions); pale, swollen nasal mucosa; oropharynx clear except for postnasal drip; + periorbital edema; + allergic shiners; + allergic crease

2. Diabetes Group

    Subjective parameters: Type 2 DM 10 yrs; prednisone increases her blood glucose; has had to use insulin in the past; follows the ADA diet; Glucophage 1000 mg BID 5 yrs

Continued

       Objective parameters: 5′1″; 180 lbs.; random fingerstick glucose 150 mg/dl; HbA$_{1C}$ 6%
          5 months ago

3. Obesity Group
    Subjective parameters: None.
    Objective parameters: 5′1″; 180 lbs.

4. Influenza Vaccine Group
    Subjective parameters: Last influenza vaccine 4 yrs ago.
    Objective parameters: None.

Step 3. Assess the parameters and determine the specific patient problems.
    Allergy Group Assessment: The patient has uncontrolled severe seasonal allergic rhinitis.
    Diabetes Group Assessment: The patient has poorly controlled type 2 diabetes mellitus.
    Obesity Group Assessment: The patient is obese.
    Influenza Group Assessment: The patient has not received the influenza vaccine for several
       years despite being at high risk for influenza.

Problem Prioritization

Step 1. Identify active patient problems.
    Seasonal allergic rhinitis
    Type 2 diabetes mellitus
    Obesity
    At risk for influenza
Step 2. Identify inactive patient problems.
    None
Step 3. Rank the problems.
    The patient's active problems that need immediate therapeutic intervention include the
       following:
    Seasonal allergic rhinitis
    The patient's active problems requiring less immediate therapeutic intervention include
       the following:
       Type 2 diabetes mellitus
       Obesity
       At risk for influenza
    The patient has no inactive problems.
    Of the patient's active problems, her seasonal allergic rhinitis is causing her the most
       immediate discomfort; interventions are needed to improve the quality of her life. Her
       type 2 diabetes mellitus and obesity are active problems, but both are stable and do not
       need immediate intervention. Her diabetes and work environment place her at risk of
       influenza, but the vaccine will not be available until later in the fall or early winter.
       Therefore the prioritized patient problem list for this patient is as follows:
       1. Seasonal Allergic Rhinitis
       2. Type 2 Diabetes Mellitus
       3. Obesity
       4. At Risk for Influenza

Selection of Specific Therapeutic Regimens

Step 1. Create a list of therapeutic options.
    Problem 1—*Seasonal Allergic Rhinitis*
    • Antihistamines
      • Systemic, nonsedating (cetirizine, fexofenadine, loratadine, desloratadine)

- Systemic, sedating (clemastine, diphenhydramine, tripelennamine, brompheniramine, chlorpheniramine, hydroxyzine, azatadine, cyproheptadine, phenindamine, azelastine)
  - Ocular (olopatadine, levocabastine)
  - Nasal (azelastine)
- Decongestants
  - Systemic (pseudoephedrine)
  - Nasal (phenylephrine, epinephrine, ephedrine, naphazoline, xylometazoline, tetrahydrozoline, oxymetazoline)
- Corticosteroids
  - Systemic (prednisone, cortisone, dexamethasone)
  - Nasal (beclomethasone, budesonide, flunisolide, fluticasone, triamcinolone)
- Anticholinergics, nasal (ipratropium bromide)

Problem 2—*Type 2 Diabetes Mellitus*

- Drugs that increase insulin release (sulfonylureas [glipizide, glyburide], meglitinides [repaglinide])
- Drugs that increase insulin responsiveness (biguanides [metformin], thiazolidinediones [rosiglitazone, pioglitazone])
- Drugs that modify intestinal carbohydrate absorption (alpha-glucosidase inhibitors [acarbose, miglitol])
- Exogenous insulin

Problem 3—*Obesity*

- Sympathomimetics (phentermine, diethylpropion, ephedra, sibutramine)
- Drugs that inhibit fat absorption (orlistat)

Problem 4—*At Risk for Influenza*

- Influenza vaccine
- Oral antivirals (amantadine, rimantadine, zanamivir, oseltamivir)

Step 2. Eliminate therapeutic options based on the comparative effectiveness of the drugs, suitability of the drug for the patient, effectiveness of past treatment regimens, cost of therapy, formulary restrictions, and ability of the patient to comply with the proposed regimen.

Problem 1—*Seasonal Allergic Rhinitis:* The recommended treatment for severe seasonal allergic rhinitis consists of a nasal corticosteroid plus an oral nonsedating antihistamine with or without an oral decongestant; short courses of oral corticosteroids may be required. The patient has nasal, ocular, and systemic symptoms. Therefore eliminate single-drug therapy with an ocular or nasal drug. Although the patient has not had an adequate trial of nasal cromolyn sodium, it is unlikely to be a effective for severe SAR. Therefore eliminate cromolyn. The patient feels that nonsedating antihistamines are ineffective but experiences dose-limiting side effects with sedating antihistamines. Antihistamines are more effective if taken regularly and the patient cannot tolerate the sedating antihistamines. Therefore eliminate the sedating antihistamines. Nasal decongestants are not intended for long-term use. Therefore eliminate nasal decongestants. Systemic decongestants may elevate blood sugars in patients with diabetes and are to be used with caution. The patient is not congested. Therefore eliminate systemic decongestants.

Problem 2—*Type 2 Diabetes Mellitus:* The recommended treatment for type 2 diabetes consists of diet, exercise, and oral hypoglycemics; some patients require short-term or long-term insulin. The drugs that increase insulin release are most effective for patients with normal weight or just a little overweight; the patient is markedly obese. Therefore eliminate the drugs that increase insulin release. The drugs that increase insulin

Continued

sensitivity are expensive, often cause weight gain, and are no more effective than biguanides alone or in combination.

Therefore eliminate the drugs that increase insulin sensitivity. Drugs that modify intestinal carbohydrate absorption have additive effects when combined with other oral hypoglycemics but are associated with significant gastrointestinal side effects (flatulence, diarrhea), so do not consider at this time. The patient has good long-term control of her diabetes, so do not consider insulin unless she is going to take oral corticosteroids.

Problem 3—*Obesity:* Dietary intervention and exercise are considered first-line treatments for obesity; pharmacologic intervention is not indicated at this time. Therefore do not consider drug therapy at this time.

Problem 4—*At Risk for Influenza:* Vaccination is the most effective method to reduce the risk of influenza. The oral antivirals are indicated for either the treatment of influenza or prevention of influenza in high-risk patients during the influenza season. Therefore eliminate the oral antivirals. The vaccine composition varies annually, but there are no other immunization alternatives.

Step 3. Select an appropriate therapeutic regimen, including drug, dosage, route, duration of therapy, and rationale.

Problem 1—*Seasonal Allergic Rhinitis:* Given the patient's diabetes mellitus and past history of requiring insulin when taking prednisone and antihistamine-associated drowsiness, a conservative initial approach is best. Once-daily therapy may improve patient adherence. Initiate therapy with a nasal corticosteroid and a nonsedating antihistamine. There is little difference among the marketed nasal corticosteroids except for fluticasone, which is better absorbed than other nasal corticosteroids. Aqueous dosage formulations may cause less nasal mucosa irritation than other dosage formulations. Initiate therapy with triamcinolone acetonide (Nasacort AQ) two sprays (220 μg) in each nostril once daily. There is little difference among the marketed nonsedating antihistamines except for cetirizine, which is more sedating than other nonsedating antihistamines. Initiate therapy with loratadine (Claritin) 10 mg once daily on an empty stomach. Advise the patient to avoid outdoor activities and to keep her car and house windows closed. Return to clinic in 2 weeks to evaluate effectiveness of regimen.

Problem 2—*Type 2 Diabetes Mellitus:* The patient's diabetes mellitus is well controlled on her current regimen. Continue metformin (Glucophage) 1000 mg BID. Continue the ADA diet, but reduce the number of calories (see obesity plan following). Encourage moderate exercise.

Problem 3—*Obesity:* The patient is obese (BMI 35 kg/m²). She is at high risk of cardiovascular complications. The goal of therapy is to lose 0.5-1 kg per week for the first 3 months. Although drug therapy could be initiated (her BMI is >30 kg/m²), the conservative approach is to try a few months of dietary restrictions and moderate exercise. Advise the patient to reduce her caloric intake to 1200 kcal/day and to start a walking program with a target of 30 minutes 5 days a week. Encourage the patient to find a "diet buddy" or join a weight loss support group.

Problem 4—*At Risk for Influenza:* Schedule the influenza vaccine for November.

Step 4. Identify alternative therapeutic regimens.

Problem 1—*Seasonal Allergic Rhinitis:* The patient may need a short course of oral corticosteroids if her symptoms have not improved after a 2-week trial of nasal corticosteroids and nonsedating antihistamine. Consider a 10-day course of prednisone (40 mg/day on days 1 & 2, 30 mg/day on days 3 & 4, 20 mg/day on days 5 & 6, 10 mg/day on days 7 & 8, 5 mg/day on days 9 & 10). Insulin may need to be added if prednisone is prescribed.

Problem 2—*Type 2 Diabetes Mellitus:* If prednisone is added to her regimen, instruct the patient to check her blood sugars four times a day and to treat elevated blood glucose with short-acting regular human insulin (no insulin if glucose is <140 mg/dl, 2 units of insulin if glucose is 140-200 mg/dl, 3 units of insulin if glucose is 201-300 mg/dl, 10 units of insulin if glucose is 301-400 mg/dl, and 12 units of insulin if glucose is >400 mg/dl); instruct the patient to call the clinic if her blood glucose is >400 mg/dl.

Problem 3—*Obesity:* Consider adding orlistat (Xenical) 120 mg TID with meals containing fat (during or up to 1 hour after the meal) if the patient has not lost weight after several months of diet and exercise. Consider sibutramine (Meridia) 10 mg once daily long term if she is not taking any sympathomimetic decongestants.

Problem 4—*At Risk for Influenza:* If the patient is not vaccinated and gets influenza, recommend oseltamivir (Tamiflu) 75 mg BID × 5 days if therapy can be initiated within 48 hours of the onset of symptoms to reduce the severity and duration of symptoms.

Initial Treatment Regimen

Consideration of all patient problems and therapeutic issues results in the following initial treatment regimen:

Avoid outdoor activities. Keep car and house windows closed.

1200 kcal/day ADA diet.

Start a walking program with a target of 30 minutes 5 days a week.

Schedule the influenza vaccine for November.

Return to clinic in 2 weeks for reassessment.

Drugs:

triamcinolone acetonide (Nasacort AQ) two sprays (220 µg) in each nostril once daily

loratadine (Claritin) 10 mg once daily

metformin (Glucophage) 1000 mg BID

SELF-ASSESSMENT QUESTIONS

1. Which one of the following is not a component of the planning process?
   a. Problem identification
   b. Problem prioritization
   c. Selection of specific initial and alternative treatment regimens
   d. Development of an integrated monitoring plan
   e. Patient counseling

2. Which one of the following is not a step involved in the identification of patient problems?
   a. Identification of subjective and objective patient parameters
   b. Creation of a working list of all patient parameters
   c. Prioritization of patient parameters
   d. Creation of sets of related problems
   e. Determination of each specific patient problem

3. Which one of the following is a subjective parameter?
   a. Serum creatinine
   b. Weight
   c. Height
   d. Dysuria
   e. Peak expiratory flow rate

4. Which one of the following is not a subjective parameter?
   a. Anxiety
   b. Indigestion
   c. Respiratory rate
   d. Insomnia
   e. Pain

5. Which one of the following is an objective parameter?
   a. Blurred vision
   b. Temperature
   c. Headache
   d. Tinnitus
   e. Fatigue

6. Which one of the following is not an objective parameter?
   a. Vertigo
   b. Urine output
   c. Bilirubin
   d. Hemoglobin
   e. Ejection fraction

7. A patient arrives in the emergency room with a serious head injury. Laboratory tests identify mild hyperlipidemia. The patient is S/P a hernia repair. Which of the following is an appropriate prioritization of the patient's problems?

	Problem #1	Problem #2	Problem #3
a.	Head injury	Hyperlipidemia	S/P hernia repair
b.	S/P hernia repair	Hyperlipidemia	Head injury
c.	Hyperlipidemia	S/P hernia repair	Head injury
d.	Hyperlipidemia	Head injury	S/P hernia repair
e.	Head injury	S/P hernia repair	Hyperlipidemia

8. A patient arrives at the medication refill clinic requesting a refill of her antihypertensive medication. She states that "It is hard to get around because my feet have been so swollen." Physical examination reveals bilateral 4+ pitting edema to the knees, scattered crackles in all lung fields, jugular venous distention, and a displaced point of maximal impulse. Blood pressure is 120/78 mm Hg. She has a penicillin allergy. Which of the following is an appropriate prioritization of the patient's problems?

	Problem #1	Problem #2	Problem #3
a.	Hypertension	Penicillin allergy	Congestive heart failure
b.	Hypertension	Congestive heart failure	Penicillin allergy
c.	Congestive heart failure	Hypertension	Penicillin allergy
d.	Congestive heart failure	Penicillin allergy	Hypertension
e.	Penicillin allergy	Congestive heart failure	Hypertension

9. Which of the following is not a step in the selection of specific therapeutic regimens?
   a. Creation of a list of therapeutic options for each problem
   b. Selection of an appropriate therapeutic regimen for each problem
   c. Identification of alternative regimens
   d. Creation of a monitoring plan and monitoring of the patient
   e. Identification of objective and subjective patient parameters

10. A patient with a dry, hacking cough asks the pharmacist to recommend a cough medication. The pharmacist, who does not know the patient, recommends a popular nonprescription cough suppressant without checking the patient's medication profile. What error did the pharmacist commit?

   a. The pharmacist should have considered other patient problems.
   b. The pharmacist should have recommended an expectorant.
   c. The pharmacist should have advised the patient to see a physician.
   d. The pharmacist should have recommended a decongestant.
   e. The pharmacist should have obtained a prescription for a cough suppressant from the patient's doctor.

Monitoring Drug Therapies

8

CHAPTER

Learning Objectives

- Identify skills needed to monitor patients.
- List and describe each step in the monitoring process.
- Identify the four types of monitoring data included in the four-square monitoring method.
- Given specific monitoring parameters, organize patient data appropriately.

atient-focused care is a never-ending cycle of data acquisition and assessment, problem identification and prioritization, therapeutic planning, and patient monitoring (Figure 8-1). Monitoring consists of identifying, obtaining, and assessing patient-specific outcome parameters. Monitoring provides the data needed to determine whether the therapeutic regimen achieves the desired goals of therapy or whether the therapeutic regimen needs to be changed secondary to inadequate response, disease progression, patient dissatisfaction, drug allergy, or undesirable or potentially dangerous adverse drug reactions.

Expertise in a variety of skills (e.g., communication skills, physical assessment skills, math skills) and excellent pharmacotherapy and human disease databases are required to monitor patients. Pharmacists in institutional patient care facilities such as acute care hospitals or long-term care facilities have many opportunities to interact with patients and have access to extensive patient-specific laboratory and diagnostic data. Pharmacists in community pharmacy settings such as retail pharmacies or outpatient clinics interact with patients through multiple but short patient encounters over prolonged periods. Access to objective patient data in the community pharmacy setting is limited but is expected to increase as multiple patient care databases are linked.

A significant amount of data is obtained by direct patient questioning and close patient observation. Routine physical examination procedures (e.g., blood pressure, heart rate, respiratory rate; lung sounds; heart sounds; diabetic foot examination) provide important patient monitoring data with minimal equipment or patient invasiveness. More comprehensive physical assessment skills (e.g., neurologic examination, funduscopic examination) may be necessary for monitoring more complex therapeutic regimens.

The amount of patient data can be extensive. For example, ambulatory patients may self-monitor blood sugar or peak expiratory flow rate several times a day. In some patient care settings (e.g., intensive care units), the patient's blood pressure

Patient-Focused Care Cycle

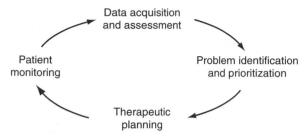

Figure 8-1
The Patient-Focused Care Cycle.
Patient-focused care is a never-ending cycle of data acquisition and assessment, problem identification and prioritization, therapeutic planning, and patient monitoring.

and electrocardiogram are monitored continuously. It is impossible to collect and assess such large masses of data. Therefore patient monitoring has to be a selective targeted process. Monitoring consists of selecting and assessing specific data for targeted outcomes. This chapter introduces a structured process and approach to monitoring patient response to drug therapy.

PROCESS

Monitoring is an organized and dynamic process (Box 8-1). The initial drug monitoring plan is developed when the initial therapeutic plan is created. It is then modified according to patient response.

STEP 1—SET THERAPEUTIC GOALS
Determine specific goals and outcomes of therapy before doing any other planning. Set specific goals for each patient problem and for the overall therapeutic outcome in general. When setting therapeutic goals, consider long-term goals such as the impact of the therapeutic regimen on the patient's quality of life and survival. For example, a long-term weight reduction plan is not appropriate for a patient with a short life expectancy. Select target therapeutic ranges for all objective parameters (e.g., systolic blood pressure between 110 and 130 mm Hg; serum potassium between 3.5 and 4.5

BOX 8-1

The Monitoring Process

Step 1 Set therapeutic goals.
Step 2 Determine patient- and drug-specific monitoring parameters.
Step 3 Integrate the monitoring plan.
Step 4 Obtain data.
Step 5 Assess the response to therapy.

mEq/L; weight between 55 and 60 kg) and identify specific target toxic outcome parameters (e.g., heart rate <50 BPM, plasma phenytoin concentration >20 mg/L). Select specific subjective outcomes for all subjective parameters (e.g., sleeping through the night without wheezing; no nocturnal leg cramps; anorexia).

Consider the severity of disease and the acuity or chronicity of therapy when setting therapeutic goals. For example, consider the differences in the goals of insulin therapy for a young patient with newly diagnosed insulin-dependent diabetes mellitus and an elderly patient with a 50-year history of insulin-dependent diabetes mellitus and significant cardiovascular and peripheral vascular disease. Evidence suggests that tight control of blood sugar levels may delay the onset and decrease the severity of the complications of diabetes. Therefore the target blood sugar level for the young patient with newly diagnosed diabetes is lower and includes a more narrow acceptable range than for the elderly patient with diabetes and long-standing disease who has already developed complications from the disease and is at risk from hypoglycemic-related falls.

STEP 2—DETERMINE PATIENT- AND DRUG-SPECIFIC MONITORING PARAMETERS

All medication regimens have two possible outcomes:
1. The medication regimen provides the expected therapeutic benefit for the patient.
2. The medication regimen does not provide the expected therapeutic benefit or is otherwise harmful to the patient.

Each outcome is assessed by questioning the patient (subjective data) and obtaining quantifiable data (objective data), giving four distinct types of monitoring data:
1. *Subjective-Therapeutic*—subjective data for assessing whether the medication regimen provides the expected therapeutic outcome
2. *Subjective-Toxic*—subjective data for assessing whether the medication regimen does not provide the expected therapeutic outcome or is otherwise harmful to the patient
3. *Objective-Therapeutic*—objective data for assessing whether the medication regimen provides the expected therapeutic outcome
4. *Objective-Toxic*—objective data for assessing whether the medication regimen does not provide the expected therapeutic outcome or is otherwise harmful to the patient

Visualize the four sets of monitoring data as four subdivisions of a large square (the four-square method) (Figure 8-2). Each subdivision represents one of the four types of monitoring data (i.e., subjective-therapeutic, subjective-toxic, objective-therapeutic, and objective-toxic data); the large square represents the complete monitoring plan. The four-square method is used to create drug-specific monitoring plans (i.e., complete one large square for each drug in a patient's medication regimen) or to create an integrated monitoring plan encompassing all the drugs in the patient's therapeutic regimen (i.e., integrate data from multiple drug-specific squares into one large square).

Consider the disease and disease-specific pharmacotherapeutics when selecting monitoring parameters. Patient symptoms will diminish or resolve if the medication achieves the expected outcome. Identify current patient symptoms and determine the target response (e.g., decreased pain, increased exercise tolerance, less shortness of breath with exertion). Identify current abnormal objective abnormalities and

Subjective-Therapeutic	Objective-Therapeutic
Subjective-Toxic	Objective-Toxic

Figure 8-2
Organization of Monitoring Parameters (The Four-Square Method).
Subjective-therapeutic monitoring parameters are subjective data for the expected therapeutic outcome.
Subjective-toxic monitoring parameters are subjective data indicating therapeutic failure or harm to the patient.
Objective-therapeutic monitoring parameters are objective data for the expected therapeutic outcome.
Objective-toxic monitoring parameters are objective data indicating therapeutic failure or harm to the patient.

determine the target response (e.g., decrease weight to 70 kg, increase FEV_1 15%, decrease heart rate to >50 BPM but <80 BPM). If the medication produces the expected targeted response, the abnormal monitoring parameters will return to normal or at least approach acceptable outcomes. Consider the potential adverse effects attributed to the specific medication and identify subjective and objective parameters that identify the adverse effects. For example, theophylline irritates the gastrointestinal tract and stimulates the heart. Ask the patient about his or her appetite and check for tachycardia.

Select appropriate subjective and objective monitoring parameters and record the monitoring parameters in the appropriate subdivision of the large square. Complete a four-square for each medication in the therapeutic regimen. This approach not only provides the pharmacist with an organized and thorough monitoring plan but also reminds the pharmacist of the relationships among the types of monitoring data and the reasons for evaluating specific parameters.

STEP 3—INTEGRATE THE MONITORING PLAN

No integration is required if the patient is receiving just one medication. However, most patients receive multiple drugs; therefore the individual medication monitoring plans must be integrated into one master monitoring plan. One way to integrate the monitoring plan is to create a master list of subjective and objective monitoring parameters collated from each of the individual medication monitoring plans, noting all the reasons for monitoring any given parameter. For example, heart rate may be an objective monitoring parameter for the therapeutic and toxic response to digoxin, the therapeutic response to procainamide, and the toxic response to theophylline. To monitor the heart rate, the pharmacist needs to measure or look up the heart rate response only once; however, the monitoring plan documents all the reasons why heart rate is being monitored.

STEP 4—OBTAIN DATA

Once the monitoring plan is created, monitor the patient's response to therapy. Interview the patient or caregiver for subjective data. Obtain objective data from the patient's medical record, bedside flow sheets, and laboratory reports.

Monitoring frequency depends on the acuteness and severity of the illness and the risks associated with the specific drug therapy. For example, patients receiving experimental combination drug therapy for the treatment of cancer need to be monitored more acutely and frequently than do patients receiving daily aspirin therapy for the prevention of cardiovascular disease. Ambulatory patients with relatively stable disease may need to be monitored as infrequently as every few months, whereas critically ill patients may need to be monitored continuously.

Document the monitoring data in organized, easily assessable formats. Flow sheets work well for documenting objective data; brief sequential serial notes work well for documenting subjective data. Most pharmacists prefer to create their own customized monitoring forms that provide a structured format for the organization of practice-specific data. Some pharmacists use institution-specific monitoring forms

SCHEDULED MEDICATIONS

Patient:		ID Number:		Physician:							
Drug Allergies/Adverse Reactions:											
Diagnosis:											
Start	Stop	Medication Dose, Route, Schedule									

Figure 8-3
Scheduled Medications Flow Sheet.
Example of a flow sheet for monitoring scheduled medications.

PRN MEDICATIONS

Patient:		ID Number:		Physician:								
Drug Allergies/Adverse Reactions:												
Diagnosis:												
Start	Stop	Medication Dose, Route, Schedule										

Figure 8-4
"As-Needed" (PRN) Medications Flow Sheet.
Example of a flow sheet for monitoring "as-needed" (PRN) medications.

that have been developed and agreed on by consensus. Figures 8-3 and 8-4 are examples of medication flow sheets and Figures 8-5 through 8-7 are examples of objective data flow sheets. Some pharmacists prefer to use commercially available patient tracking software published for personal data assistants (PDAs).

STEP 5—ASSESS THE RESPONSE TO THERAPY
Assess the subjective and objective data to determine the patient's response to therapy. Look for isolated abnormalities as well as for trends. Recognizing trends is as important as recognizing individual abnormalities. For example, a slowly decreasing serum platelet count is as important as a single hypoglycemic reaction to a larger-than-necessary dose of insulin.

There is no need to change the therapeutic regimen if the medication regimen achieves the desired outcomes. However, the therapeutic regimen must be changed if it does not achieve the desired therapeutic outcome or if it is associated with intolerable or potentially dangerous adverse effects (Box 8-2). Dosages may be increased or decreased; drugs may be deleted or added to the regimen. Make the appropriate changes to the therapeutic regimen, modify the monitoring plan, and continue the patient-focused care cycle.

APPLICATION AND INTEGRATION

The case study on p. 178 illustrates the patient-focused care cycle.

	Time and Date																		
Sodium																			
Potassium																			
Chloride																			
CO_2 content																			
BUN																			
Creatinine																			
Glucose																			
Calcium																			
Magnesium																			
Phosphorus																			
Uric acid																			
Bilirubin, total																			
Bilirubin, direct																			
Bilirubin, delta																			
Protein, total																			
Albumin																			
Globulin																			
LDH																			
AST																			
ALT																			
AP																			
CPK																			
Amylase																			
Ammonia																			
RBCs																			
Reticulocytes																			
Hemoglobin																			
Hematocrit																			
ESR																			
WBCs																			
PMNs																			
Bands																			
Lymphocytes																			
Eosinophils																			
Other																			
Platelets																			
PT/INR																			
PTT																			
ABG																			
Fio_2																			
pH																			
$Paco_2$																			
Pao_2																			
Bicarbonate																			
Base excess																			
Sao_2																			

Figure 8-5
Laboratory Flow Sheet.
Example of a flow sheet for monitoring laboratory data.

	Time and Date														
Blood Pressure															
Heart Rate															
Cardiac Output															
Cardiac Index															
MAP															
RAP															
RVP															
RVP, systolic															
RVP, diastolic															
PAP, mean															
PAP, systolic															
PAP, diastolic															
PAOP, mean															
SVR															
PVR															
Cao_2															
Cvo_2															

Figure 8-6
Hemodynamics Flow Sheet.
Example of a flow sheet for monitoring hemodynamic data.

Date	Site	Gram's Stain	Organism(s)	Susceptibilities	
				Sensitive	Resistant

Figure 8-7
Microbiology Flow Sheet.
Example of a flow sheet for monitoring microbiology data.

BOX 8-2

Guidelines for Altering Drug Therapy

If the regimen is ineffective, change the drug if:
 1. The patient received an adequate trial of the drug.
 2. The patient received an adequate dosage of the drug.
 3. The patient adhered to the prescribed or recommended regimen.
If the regimen is associated with life-threatening side effects, discontinue the drug.
If the patient will not comply with the prescribed or recommended regimen because of unacceptable side effects, discontinue the drug.
If the patient has non-life-threatening side effects and is willing to continue the drug, minimize the side effects:
 1. Modify the dosage.
 2. Change drug administration times.

▪ *Case Study* ▪

JC, a 69-year-old white male with a diagnosis of right- and left-sided congestive heart failure, complains of swollen feet, shortness of breath when walking more than half a block, nonproductive cough that is worse at night, and occasional leg cramps. He gained 30 pounds over the past 3 months and notes that all his clothes are too tight. He props himself up with three pillows when sleeping. The goal of therapy is to improve the patient's quality of life by improving cardiac function and controlling symptoms. His new medication regimen includes digoxin (Lanoxin) 0.25 mg daily, furosemide (Lasix) 40 mg daily, captopril (Capoten) 25 mg three times daily, and potassium chloride (Slow-K) 8 mEq three times daily.

Digoxin Monitoring Parameters (Figure 8-8)

Subjective-Therapeutic Monitoring Parameters—The patient's symptoms will diminish or resolve if digoxin therapy provides the expected therapeutic benefit of improved cardiac function.

Subjective-Toxic Monitoring Parameters—The patient's symptoms will not improve and may worsen if digoxin therapy does not provide the expected therapeutic benefit and the patient may experience a variety of annoying or potentially harmful side effects from digoxin therapy.

Objective-Therapeutic Monitoring Parameters—A variety of laboratory and other tests are used to monitor improvement in cardiac function. Improved cardiac function may not be immediately evident after initiation of treatment but may be apparent with long-term drug therapy.

Objective-Toxic Monitoring Parameters—A variety of laboratory and other tests are used to monitor for lack of improvement in cardiac function or potentially harmful side effects from digoxin therapy.

Furosemide Monitoring Parameters (Figure 8-9)

Subjective-Therapeutic Monitoring Parameters—The patient's symptoms will decrease or resolve if furosemide therapy improves cardiac function by decreasing intravascular volume.

Subjective-Therapeutic	Objective-Therapeutic
↓ Swelling of feet Looser-fitting clothing ↓ SOB and DOE ↑ Exercise tolerance Sleeps with fewer pillows ↓ Cough	↓ Heart size on CXR ↓ Edema on CXR ↓ Weight ↑ Ejection fraction Improved R-wave progression Normalization of R-S ↓ T-wave inversion
Subjective-Toxic	**Objective-Toxic**
↑ Swelling of feet Tighter-fitting clothing ↑ SOB and DOE ↓ Exercise tolerance More problems sleeping ↑ Cough ↓ Appetite Nausea Vomiting Halos around lights Yellowish visual tinting Abdominal discomfort Palpitations Weakness Lethargy Agitation or disorientation	↑ Heart size on CXR ↑ Edema on CXR ↑ Weight ↓ Ejection fraction Poor R-wave progression Abnormal R-S ↑ T-wave inversion VPDs Cardiac arrhythmias Serum digoxin >2 ng/ml ↓ Heart rate <50 BPM ↓ SBP <100 mm Hg ↓ DBP <60 mm Hg

Figure 8-8
Digoxin Monitoring Plan.
Example of subjective and objective monitoring parameters for digoxin.

Subjective-Toxic Monitoring Parameters—The patient's symptoms will not improve and may worsen if furosemide therapy does not provide the expected therapeutic benefit. The patient also may experience a variety of annoying or potentially harmful side effects from furosemide therapy.

Objective-Therapeutic Monitoring Parameters—A variety of laboratory and other tests are used to monitor improvement in the fluid overload status of the patient. Some improvement in cardiac function may occur as a result of diuretic therapy.

Objective-Toxic Monitoring Parameters—A variety of laboratory and other tests are used to monitor for lack of improvement in cardiac function or potentially harmful side effects from furosemide therapy.

Continued

Subjective-Therapeutic	Objective-Therapeutic
↓ Swelling of feet Looser-fitting clothing ↓ SOB and DOE Able to sleep with fewer pillows ↓ Cough	↓ Heart size on CXR ↓ Edema on CXR ↓ Weight ↑ Ejection fraction Improved R-wave progression Normalization of R-S ↓ T-wave inversion
Subjective-Toxic	**Objective-Toxic**
↑ Swelling of feet Tighter-fitting clothing ↑ SOB and DOE More problems sleeping ↑ Cough Muscle cramps Dry mouth Thirst Dizziness Upset stomach Weakness Palpitations Lethargy Confusion	↑ Heart size on CXR ↑ Edema on CXR ↑ Weight ↓ Ejection fraction Poor R-wave progression Abnormal R-S ↑ T-wave inversion ↓ Serum potassium ↑ Serum glucose ↑ Serum uric acid ↑ Serum BUN/creatinine ratio ↑ Serum BUN ↑ Serum creatinine ↓ Blood pressure ↑ Heart rate U wave or flattened T wave

Figure 8-9
Furosemide Monitoring Plan.
Example of subjective and objective monitoring parameters for furosemide.

Captopril Monitoring Parameters (Figure 8-10)

Subjective-Therapeutic Monitoring Parameters—The patient's symptoms will decrease or resolve if captopril therapy provides the expected therapeutic benefit of improved cardiac function.

Subjective-Toxic Monitoring Parameters—The patient's symptoms will not improve and may worsen if captopril therapy does not provide the expected therapeutic benefit. The

Subjective-Therapeutic	Objective-Therapeutic
↓ Swelling of feet Looser-fitting clothing ↓ SOB and DOE ↑ Exercise tolerance Able to sleep with fewer pillows ↓ Cough	↓ Heart size on CXR ↓ Edema on CXR ↓ Weight ↑ Ejection fraction Improved R-wave progression Normalization of R-S ↓ T-wave inversion
Subjective-Toxic	**Objective-Toxic**
↑ Swelling of feet Tighter-fitting clothing ↑ SOB and DOE ↓ Exercise tolerance More problems sleeping Persistent dry cough Dizziness Itching Maculopapular or morbilliform rash Dysgeusia	↑ Heart size on CXR ↑ Edema on CXR ↑ Weight ↓ Ejection fraction Poor R-wave progression Abnormal R-S ↑ T-wave inversion Elevated temperature Eosinophilia Proteinuria ↑ Serum creatinine ↑ Serum BUN ↓ Blood pressure WBC with differential

Figure 8-10
Captopril Monitoring Plan.
Subjective and objective monitoring parameters for captopril.

patient also may experience a variety of annoying or potentially harmful side effects from captopril therapy.

Objective-Therapeutic Monitoring Parameters—A variety of laboratory and other tests are used to monitor improvement in cardiac function. Improvement in cardiac function may not be immediately evident after initiation of treatment but may be noted after long-term drug administration.

Objective-Toxic Monitoring Parameters—A variety of laboratory and other tests are used to monitor for lack of improvement in cardiac function or potentially harmful side effects from captopril therapy.   *Continued*

Subjective-Therapeutic	Objective-Therapeutic
None.	Serum potassium 3.5-5 mEq/L
Subjective-Toxic	**Objective-Toxic**
Nausea Vomiting Diarrhea Bad taste Abdominal discomfort Palpitations Lethargy Weakness Muscle cramps	Serum potassium <3.5 mEq/L Flattened T wave Widened Q-R-S complex Peaked T waves Flattened or inverted T waves U waves

Figure 8-11
Potassium Chloride Monitoring Plan.
Example of subjective and objective monitoring parameters for potassium chloride.

Potassium Chloride Monitoring Parameters (Figure 8-11)
   Subjective-Therapeutic Monitoring Parameters—The patient is receiving supplemental
      potassium to prevent hypokalemia resulting from the furosemide therapy. Because this is
      preventive therapy, no subjective parameters are available to evaluate the desired out-
      come of supplemental potassium therapy.
   Subjective-Toxic Monitoring Parameters—The patient may develop hypokalemia if potas-
      sium supplementation is inadequate. Conversely, if potassium supplementation is exces-
      sive, the patient may experience symptoms of hyperkalemia.
   Objective-Therapeutic Monitoring Parameters—The goal of therapy is to maintain an
      appropriate serum potassium level with supplemental therapy.
   Objective-Toxic Monitoring Parameters—Objective monitoring parameters for supple-
      mental potassium therapy are limited.

Integrated Monitoring Plan (Box 8-3 and Box 8-4)
The drugs in the therapeutic regimen are prescribed for the management of congestive heart
failure. Therefore a great deal of duplication occurs among the monitoring plans. However, the
pharmacist needs to know the multiple reasons for monitoring each parameter. For example,

BOX 8-3

Integrated Subjective Monitoring Plan for Digoxin, Furosemide, Captopril, and Potassium Chloride

---

SUBJECTIVE THERAPEUTIC MONITORING PARAMETERS
General: Looser-fitting clothing; able to sleep with fewer pillows
Pulmonary: ↓ SOB and DOE; ↑ exercise tolerance; ↓ cough
Extremities: ↓ Swelling of feet

SUBJECTIVE TOXIC MONITORING PARAMETERS
General: Tighter-fitting clothing; more problems sleeping; weakness; lethargy; agitation or
  disorientation; confusion; dizziness
Vision: Halos around lights; yellowish visual tint
Pulmonary: ↑ SOB and DOE; ↓ exercise tolerance; ↑ cough, persistent dry cough
Cardiac: Palpitations
Gastrointestinal: Dry mouth; thirst; ↓ appetite; nausea; vomiting; abdominal discomfort;
  upset stomach; diarrhea; dysgeusia
Extremities: ↑ Swelling of feet; muscle cramps
Skin: Itching; maculopapular or morbilliform rash

DOE, Dyspnea on exestion; SOB, shortness of breath.

BOX 8-4

Integrated Objective Monitoring Plan for Digoxin, Furosemide, Captopril, and Potassium Chloride

---

OBJECTIVE THERAPEUTIC MONITORING PARAMETERS
↓ Weight
CXR: ↓ Heart size, ↓ edema
↑ Ejection fraction
ECG: Improved R-wave progression; normalization of S-R; ↓ T-wave inversion
Labs: Serum potassium 3.5-5 mEq/L

OBJECTIVE TOXIC MONITORING PARAMETERS
↑ Weight
CXR: ↑ Heart size, ↑ edema
↓ Ejection fraction
ECG: Poor R-wave progression; abnormal R-S on ECG; ↑ T-wave inversion; VPDs;
  arrhythmias; U waves or flat or inverted T waves; flattened P waves; widened QRS
  complex; peaked T waves
Serum digoxin > 2 ng/ml
Vitals: ↓ Heart rate; ↓ blood pressure; ↑ temperature
Labs: ↑ Serum potassium; ↑ serum glucose; ↑ serum uric acid; ↑ serum BUN/Cr ratio;
  ↑ serum BUN; ↑ serum creatinine; eosinophilia; proteinuria; WBC with differential

BUN, Blood urea nitrogen; CXR, chest radiograph; ECG, electrocardiogram; VPD, ventricular
premature deplorization; WBC, white blood cell count.

blood pressure is an important therapeutic and toxic monitoring parameter for several of the drugs in the medication regimen.

Monitor the patient frequently (e.g., weekly) for initial response to therapy then less frequently (e.g., every 6 months) as the patient's condition stabilizes. Therapeutic monitoring is an ongoing process. Modify the therapeutic regimen and monitoring plan according to the patient's response.

SELF-ASSESSMENT QUESTIONS

1. Which of the following are needed to monitor a patient's response to drug therapy?
   a. Knowledge of pharmacotherapeutics
   b. Knowledge of pathophysiology
   c. Communication skills
   d. Physical assessment skills
   e. All of the above

2. Which of the following is the first step in the monitoring process?
   a. Monitor the response to therapy.
   b. Assess the response to therapy.
   c. Set therapeutic goals.
   d. Integrate the monitoring plan.
   e. Determine specific monitoring parameters.

3. Which of the following is the last step in the monitoring process?
   a. Monitor the response to therapy.
   b. Assess the response to therapy.
   c. Set therapeutic goals.
   d. Integrate the monitoring plan.
   e. Determine specific monitoring parameters.

4. For which kind of patient is the availability of monitoring data limited?
   a. A hospitalized, critically ill patient
   b. A patient just started on insulin therapy
   c. A patient with stable, well-controlled mild hypertension
   d. A patient undergoing renal dialysis
   e. A postsurgical trauma patient

5. For which kind of patient is the largest amount of monitoring data available?
   a. A hospitalized, critically ill patient
   b. A patient just started on insulin therapy
   c. A patient with stable, well-controlled mild hypertension
   d. A patient undergoing renal dialysis
   e. A postsurgical trauma patient

6. A patient is receiving a medication associated with hypokalemia (reference range of 3.5 to 5.5 mEq/L). Which of the following is an appropriate therapeutic goal when monitoring potassium-replacement therapy?
   a. Serum potassium 4.0 mEq/L
   b. Serum potassium greater than 5.5 mEq/L
   c. Serum potassium less than 3.5 mEq/L
   d. Serum potassium 3.5 to 5.5 mEq/L
   e. Serum potassium 2.0 to 3.0 mEq/L

Refer to the following information for questions 7 through 10: A patient with pneumonia is receiving an antibiotic for treatment of acute bronchitis. The patient's symptoms include cough and fever. The antibiotic may cause diarrhea and thrombocytopenia.

7. *Decreased cough* is what type of monitoring parameter?
   a. Subjective-therapeutic
   b. Subjective-toxic
   c. Objective-therapeutic
   d. Objective-toxic
   e. None of the above

8. *Decreased fever* is what type of monitoring parameter?
   a. Subjective-therapeutic
   b. Subjective-toxic
   c. Objective-therapeutic
   d. Objective-toxic
   e. None of the above

9. *Diarrhea* is what type of monitoring parameter?
   a. Subjective-therapeutic
   b. Subjective-toxic
   c. Objective-therapeutic
   d. Objective-toxic
   e. None of the above

10. *Thrombocytopenia* is what type of monitoring parameter?
   a. Subjective-therapeutic
   b. Subjective-toxic
   c. Objective-therapeutic
   d. Objective-toxic
   e. None of the above

Researching and Providing Drug Information

9

CHAPTER

Learning Objectives

- Identify the components involved in providing drug information to health care professionals and patients.
- Identify and categorize common types of drug information questions.
- List examples of questions used to clarify the initial drug information question.
- State the key to a successful search of the published literature.
- Differentiate among primary, secondary, and tertiary literature.
- State how to evaluate primary, secondary, and tertiary literature.
- Describe how to access information in textbooks, files using the AHFS numbering system, *Index Medicus*, computerized databases, and the Internet.
- List the advantages and disadvantages of using the Internet to access drug information.
- State how to evaluate Internet drug information websites.
- Describe the best way to communicate answers to drug information questions.

D issemination of information regarding medications and other pharmaceuticals is an important responsibility. Patients, physicians, nurses, and other health care professionals depend on pharmacists for accurate and timely information about medications. Pharmacists commonly answer questions about drug dosing, product availability, and drug side effects, as well as a variety of other drug-related issues (Box 9-1).

To respond effectively to drug information questions, pharmacists need good communication skills, knowledge of literature resources and ways to access them, and the ability to evaluate published information. Some questions can be answered by relying on previously acquired knowledge; other questions require a search and assessment of the published medical and pharmacy literature.

PROCESS

The components involved in the provision of drug information include determining the primary question, developing an appropriate search strategy, locating appropriate sources of information if the question cannot be answered from previously acquired knowledge, assessing the available information, and providing a verbal or written response to the question.

BOX 9-1

Types of Drug Information Questions

ADVERSE DRUG REACTIONS
Adverse reactions
Allergies
Teratogenicity
Toxicology

DOSING
Age-specific dosing
Dosing in altered organ function (liver, renal)
Indication-specific dosing

DRUG ADMINISTRATION
Commercial dosage form alterations (crushing, dissolving)
Drug administration methods
Product preparation (reconstitution, admixing, compounding)
Compatibility, stability, and storage
Timing (with or without food or enteral products)

DRUG INTERACTIONS
Drug-disease
Drug-drug
Drug-food
Drug-laboratory
Drug-nutrient

INDICATIONS AND THERAPEUTIC USE
Approved drugs
Investigational drugs
Unapproved drugs

POISONINGS AND TOXICOLOGY
Signs and symptoms
Treatment

PRODUCT-SPECIFIC CONCERNS
Constituents (sugars, dyes, adjuvants, alcohol)
Formulations
Identification
Storage

MISCELLANEOUS
Drug use during pregnancy and lactation
Pharmacoeconomics
Product-specific assays
Veterinary drug information

DETERMINING THE PRIMARY QUESTION

Most questions arise as the result of a patient-specific problem; however, questions often are presented initially as broad-based theoretical issues. For example, a physician may ask for the incidence of ceftriaxone allergic reactions when in fact the actual question is whether ceftriaxone is the cause of an otherwise unexplained neutropenia in a specific patient. Patients may have the same difficulty phrasing questions as do health care professionals. For example, many patients do not understand the difference between an allergy and an adverse reaction. Patients may ask about drug allergies when they really want to know whether the medication they are taking is the cause of a specific problem such as nausea, constipation, headache, or drowsiness.

To determine the primary question, ask the person asking the question several clarifying questions. A good starting point is to ask whether the question pertains to a specific patient and if so to ask for pertinent background patient information. For example, if the question is about the possibility of an adverse reaction in a specific patient, inquire about the nature of the suspected problem and obtain details about the patient's current medication regimen, including drugs, dosages, and duration of therapy. Laboratory and physical examination findings also may be important pertinent details. Questions about therapeutic options may require even more information about the patient's diagnoses and past and current medication regimens.

After the primary question and patient-specific details have been identified, rephrase and restate the question. Ask clarifying questions and exchange information until the primary question is agreed on and enough patient-specific information is known to allow for a focused search for an answer. A chart review and/or direct patient interview may be necessary to locate all pertinent background patient information.

Determine when the answer is needed and how to contact the person who asked the question. Some questions require an immediate response for an urgent patient care decision; other questions are not as urgent and can be answered later the same day or even several days later. Do not assume that every question is urgent and has to be answered immediately at the expense of other responsibilities or, conversely, that every question can be put off to another day. Ask for the person's telephone or beeper number or arrange to provide the information face to face at a certain time and place such as in the clinic the next afternoon or during patient rounds later that morning.

DEVELOPING AN APPROPRIATE SEARCH STRATEGY

Searching for drug information is a complex process that requires significant thought before action. A great deal of time can be wasted by searching for information in the wrong places or by searching the online literature with inappropriate search terms. Therefore formulate a strategy for locating the answer to the question before actually searching for the answer to the question.

The key to developing an appropriate search strategy is to think about the question and match the question with the most appropriate information sources. Questions of fact, such as dosage formulations, usual dosage regimens, dosage adjustments for patients with renal and hepatic dysfunction, pharmacokinetic parameters for drugs that have been marketed for several years, and spectrum of activities of marketed antibiotics, are best answered by looking up the information in standard pharmacy textbooks such as the *American Hospital Formulary Service* (AHFS), standard electronic databases such as *Micromedex*, or personal data assistant (PDA) databases such as *A to Z Drug Facts*. Questions about investigational drugs, unapproved indications for currently marketed drugs, and unusual adverse effects and drug interactions are best answered by a thorough literature search of published medical and pharmacy literature accessed through databases such as MEDLINE.

The key to a successful search of the published literature is to identify appropriate search terms before starting the search. Terms can be identified by reading about the topic in a standard medical or pharmacy textbook or published review article or using indexing lists, such as the National Library of Medicine's *Medical Subject Headings* (MeSH), used to index key terms for the MEDLINE database. These indexing terms are generally relevant for searches of any medical- or pharmacy-related database.

Flexibility is important when searching for information. If a search does not reveal any relevant information, it may be that there is no information to be found. However, most of the time the search strategy is faulty. For example, the literature may not have been searched far enough back in time to locate older information or the search terms were not appropriate. Consider when information about a drug is most likely to have been published and try other related indexing terms before deciding that no information about the topic is available in the published literature.

CHOOSING SOURCES OF INFORMATION

Drug information is available from a variety of sources. Primary, secondary, and tertiary literature are the mainstays of drug information. Other information sources include colleagues and pharmaceutical companies. Colleagues may be excellent sources of information; however, the information may be dated or incomplete and is ordinarily without reference. A pharmaceutical company may be a good source of information about company-specific drug-related issues. Information may be obtained by contacting the company's drug information center or product manager or by making a written inquiry. However, pharmaceutical companies provide information regarding labeled indications only. Pharmaceutical companies cannot disclose confidential data, nor can they discuss other proprietary information. In addition, the pharmaceutical industry is required by law to compile and report adverse drug reaction information. If a company receives an inquiry regarding a possible adverse effect associated with one of its products, the company is obligated to obtain detailed information about the event and report it to the federal government.

Primary Literature. Primary literature, consisting of original data, research, and case reports, is published in journals, other periodicals, and collections of research presentations or other special proceedings (Box 9-2). Primary literature generally contains the most recent information available for any given topic. The amount of full-text primary literature posted directly on the Internet is growing rapidly. Many major medical journals provide subscribers access to full-text literature through the journal's website. Pharmacy and medical libraries may provide registered users access to full-text literature through bundled databases.

Although primary literature is published in many venues, the quality of the information varies greatly. No information can be accepted at face value without a complete assessment of how the information was derived. One initial judge of the quality of a journal is the impact or perceived prestige of the journal. Authors try to publish in journals that have the greatest impact on health care professionals. Therefore these journals receive a lot of submissions. The high number of submissions means that editors can select the highest-quality research with the most important results. Other general indications of quality include the overall reputation of the journal and

BOX 9-2

Common Primary Drug Information Sources

MEDICAL JOURNALS
General medical journals
  American Journal of Medicine
  Annals of Internal Medicine
  Journal of the American Medical Association
  Lancet
  New England Journal of Medicine
Specialty medical journals
  American Journal of Cardiology
  American Journal of Respiratory and Critical Care Medicine
  Blood
  Circulation
  Diabetes
  Gastroenterology
  Journal of Infectious Disease

PHARMACY AND PHARMACOLOGY JOURNALS
  American Journal of Health-System Pharmacy
  Annals of Pharmacotherapy
  Clinical Pharmacology and Therapeutics
  Hospital Pharmacy
  Journal of Clinical Pharmacology
  Pharmacotherapy

whether the journal uses a peer-review process when selecting articles to be published.

The reputation of a journal can be judged based on the citation rates for the articles contained within them. In a 1986 report on the impact of medical journals, the *New England Journal of Medicine* and *Lancet* accounted for more than one third of all the 1981 citations.[1] Other frequently cited journals included the *Annals of Internal Medicine*, the *British Medical Journal*, and the *Journal of the American Medical Association*. These are general medical journals; specialty and subspecialty journals have smaller circulations and therefore fewer citations.

Refereed articles have undergone peer review before acceptance for publication. The editors, after an initial internal review of the manuscript, ask outside experts for a thorough review of the manuscript. Peer review provides expert opinion regarding the originality of the material, validity of the data, appropriateness of the conclusions, and importance and relevance of the information.

Secondary and Tertiary Literature.   Secondary and tertiary literature consists of compiled information, including information from multiple databases, review articles published in journals, symposia published in journal supplements, and textbooks (Box 9-3). Secondary and tertiary literature comprises reviews, analyses, interpretations, opinions, assessments, and conclusions drawn from multiple sources of infor-

BOX 9-3

Common Secondary and Tertiary Drug Information Sources

PERIODICALS
Clin-Alert
Facts and Comparisons Drug Newsletter
FDA Medical Bulletin
The Medical Letter
DRUGDEX System
International Pharmaceutical Abstracts
Iowa Drug Information System
POISINDEX System
Unlisted Drugs

TEXTBOOKS
American drug index, ed 46, St Louis, 2002, Facts and Comparisons.
McEvoy GK: *AHFS drug information*, Bethesda, Md, 2002, American Society of Health-System Pharmacists.
Young LY, Koda-Kimble MA, Kradjan WA, et al (eds): *Applied therapeutics: the clinical use of drugs*, ed 7, Philadelphia, 2001, Lippincott Williams & Wilkins.
Evans WE, Schentag JJ, Jusko WJ: *Applied pharmacokinetics: principles of therapeutic drug monitoring*, ed 3, Vancouver, Wash, 1992, Applied Therapeutics.
Hansten PD, Horn PD: *Hansten and Horn managing clinically important drug interactions*, St Louis, 2002, Facts and Comparisons.
Drug facts and comparisons, ed 56, St Louis, 2001, Facts and Comparisons.
Tatro DS (ed): *Tatro's Drug interactions facts*, ed 10, St Louis, 2002, Facts and Comparisons.
Handbook of antimicrobial therapy, New Rochelle, NY, 1998, Medical Letter.
Anderson PO, Troutman WG, Knoben JE (eds): *Handbook of clinical drug data*, ed 10, Stamford, Conn, 2001, Appleton & Lange.
Trissel LA: *Handbook on injectable drugs*, ed 10, Bethesda, Md, 1998, American Society of Health System Pharmacists.
Berardi RR, DeSimone EM, Newton GD, et al (eds): *Handbook of nonprescription drugs*, ed 13, Washington, DC, 2002, American Pharmaceutical Association.
True B-L, Dreisbach RH (eds): *Dreisbach's handbook of poisoning: prevention, diagnosis, and treatment*, ed 13, London, 2001, CRC Press-Parthenon Publishers.
Braunwald E, Fauci AS, Kasper DL et al (eds): *Harrison's principles of internal medicine*, ed 15, New York, 2001, McGraw-Hill.
Parfitt K (ed): *Martindale's the extra pharmacopoeia*, ed 32, London, 1999, Royal Pharmaceutical Society.
O'Neil MJ, Smith A (eds): *Merck index: an encyclopedia of chemicals, drugs, and biologicals*, ed 13, Whitehouse Station, NJ, 2001, Merck.
Dukes MNG: *Meyler's side effects of drugs*, ed 13, New York, 1996, Elsevier.
DiPiro JT, Talbert RL, Yee GC et al (eds): *Pharmacotherapy*, ed 5, Stamford, Conn, 2002, Appleton & Lange.
Mosby's drug consult 2004, ed 14, St Louis, 2004, Mosby.
Physician's desk reference, ed 56, Montvale, NJ, 2002, Medical Economics.
Physican's desk reference for herbal medicine, ed 2, Montvale, NJ, 2000, Medical Economics.
Gennaro AR, Gennaro AL (eds): *Remington: the science and practice of pharmacy*, ed 20, Philadelphia, 2000, Lippincott Williams & Wilkins.

Continued

Common Secondary and Tertiary Drug Information Sources—cont'd

TEXTBOOKS—cont'd
USP drug information for health care professionals, ed 21, Rockville, Md, 2001, United States
   Pharmacopeia Convention.
Herfindal ET, Gourley DR: *Textbook of therapeutics,* ed 7, Baltimore, 2000, Williams & Wilkins.
United States pharmacopoeia—national formulary (USP25/NF20), Rockville, Md, 2001, Board of
   Trustees (United States Pharmacopeial Convention).

mation, including personal experience. Authorship of secondary and tertiary literature does not guarantee expertise.

The distinction between secondary and tertiary literature is indistinct. Although
compiled periodicals and abstracting services are commonly referred to as *secondary
literature* and textbooks and compendia are commonly referred to as *tertiary literature,*
overlap occurs. Secondary literature tends to be slightly more current than tertiary
literature but may not be subject to as extensive prepublication review as the tertiary
literature.

Textbooks and other published books are the least up-to-date sources of information because publication takes 2 to 3 years and the information contained in a book
is out of date by at least that length of time the moment the book is published. In
addition, the author or authors may have taken a year or more to write the text.
A several-year gap may exist between new editions of textbooks, making the information even more out of date.

Secondary and tertiary literature can be a good source of general or overview
information about a topic but cannot be relied on to provide the most up-to-date
information regarding indications, usages, mechanisms of action, adverse effects,
and drug interactions. Secondary and tertiary literature may not contain any information about investigational drugs, newly marketed drugs, uncommon side effects
and drug interactions, or new indications for previously marketed drugs.

ACCESSING PRINTED SOURCES OF INFORMATION

Printed sources of information are accessed by searching the indexes of textbooks,
locating articles in individually maintained files of journal article reprints, and
searching online bibliographic services. Many biomedical textbooks are published
electronically, accessible online or on CDs. Biomedical libraries, pharmacy libraries,
and institutional (e.g., hospital) libraries contain limited to extensive print
resources. Online resources are available in most biomedical libraries. Many
patient care areas (e.g., hospital wards, clinics, private offices) have access to online
resources.

Textbooks.   Most people are familiar with locating information using textbook
indexes. The key to locating information through textbook indexes is to look for the
precise topic and think of synonyms and related terms if the initial topic is not listed.

Individual Files.   The location of articles in individually maintained files of journal
article reprints depends on the system used to file the articles. Some pharmacists use

complex filing strategies. For example, some pharmacists set up their files using the American Hospital Formulary System (AHFS) numbering system. To locate specific topics, the searcher must be familiar with the AHFS or look up the drug topic in the AHFS book. Other pharmacists use simpler but highly individualized topic groupings based on specific disease states, organ systems, or pharmacotherapeutic categories.

Computerized Databases.   The availability of computerized databases has simplified the process of obtaining drug information and greatly expanded access to published information. Examples of health-related databases include MEDLINE (the online equivalent of *Index Medicus*), Current Contents, International Pharmaceutical Abstracts (IPA), and Cancerlit. Computerized databases can be searched by librarians as a service for health care professionals or by the end-user. End-user online searching is rapidly becoming the standard of practice as appropriately equipped computers are becoming more accessible in patient care areas, drug information centers, medical and pharmacy libraries, offices, and homes.

Online searching of computerized databases is best suited for specific drug information questions and information about recent topics. Getting a broad-based overview of complex topics is more difficult with online database searching; textbooks are better sources of this type of information. Many online databases were started in the mid-1960s and early 1970s; information dating earlier than this time usually has to be searched manually. Access to computerized databases is through public and commercial vendors. The National Library of Medicine (NLM), the creator of MEDLINE, is an example of a public vendor. Dialog Information Services and Bibliographic Retrieval Services (BRS) are examples of commercial vendors.

Two types of information are available to users of computerized databases. First, most databases provide at least the full bibliographic citation, including all authors, title, journal, year, volume number, issue number, and inclusive page numbers. Key indexing terms are listed, which may narrow the search, provide additional search terms, and suggest related topics. Second, the manuscript abstract may be provided. Some of the databases provide the full text of the manuscripts contained in the database; other databases provide the full text of a variety of pharmacy and medical textbooks. Generally, the information can be downloaded and printed on the end user's printer.

Online searching requires access to a computer, modem, communications software, and a knowledge of how to access computerized databases. Some training is required to learn to use the search programs; however, user-friendly programs requiring minimal training are available.

Online searching may be quite expensive, depending on the annual fee for access to the service and the charge for each search. The fee for each search depends on the amount of time connected to the database, amount of processing the computer must do to accomplish the search, number of characters printed, and time of day.

The Internet.   Searchable databases are limited to previously published information (e.g., studies, reviews, editorials, letters to the editor). This limit confers a certain degree of reliability but restricts access to other information. Although the availability of full-text publications is increasing, it remains limited to major medical journals. In addition, some delay (weeks to months) always occurs between publication in the print media and inclusion of the information in the database. In contrast, information posted directly on the Internet is completely unrestricted and posted very quickly after publication.

The Internet, consisting of thousands of connected computer networks, provides access to a wide array of information, including information traditionally published in newsletters, magazines, journals, newspapers, and books, as well as access to live discussion groups, sound tracks, and video images. Government health agencies, international health organizations, pharmaceutical companies, and professional organizations also post information on the Internet.[2,3] One clear advantage of the Internet is the connection of information through cross-listings and links that provide rapid access to related information on the Internet.

Access to information on the Internet requires a computer, modem, telephone line, access to a provider service, and specific networking and application software computer programs. The primary advantage of the Internet (access to a vast array of unlimited and uncontrolled information) also is its greatest disadvantage; no limits are placed on information posted on the Internet. No person or group controls the Internet, no universal indexing system is available, and no quality controls are in place. Locating information may be time-consuming and frustrating. In addition, no assurances are made as to the validity and/or reliability of the information.

Information is searched for and retrieved using search engines (e.g., Google, LookSmart, Netscape Search, Yahoo), software programs that index and search Internet resources. Search engines locate information by searching for specific terms and phrases; links between terms can be made using Boolean logic (e.g., and, or, not). Search results are displayed in ranked lists according to the degree to which the terms and topics match; specific information is located by opening and reading the content of the lists. Because search engines differ in the scope of Internet sources searched, searches with more than one search engine may disclose different information.

Locating incomplete, inaccurate, or false information on the Internet is a risk. Although sites should be assessed carefully before using the information to answer a drug information question, site quality is difficult to assess.[4] Several organizations (e.g., Health Information Technology Institute of Mitretek Sysetms,[5] Health on the Net Foundation,[6] National Center for Complementary and Alternative Medicine[7]) have proposed guides for assessing websites that offer health-related information (Box 9-4). Consider these questions before accepting information contained on any website. The Health on the Net (HON) Foundation is an example of a self-regulatory, voluntary certification system for health care websites.[6] Sites that meet HON criteria are identified by a blue-and-red HONcode seal, usually displayed on a site's home page. Government (e.g., www.fda.gov, www.nih.gov, www.nlm.nih.gov), pharmaceutical industry (e.g., GlaxoSmithKline, www.gsk.com; AstraZeneca, www.astrazeneca-us.com), professional (e.g., American Pharmacists Association, www.apha.org; American Society of Health-System Pharmacists, www.ashp.org), and academic-based (Arizona Poison and Drug Information Center, www.pharmacy.arizona.edu) websites are generally reliable drug information sources.

CRITICAL APPRAISAL OF INFORMATION SOURCES
Information from any source must be appraised critically. Evaluate all information, including textbooks, review articles published in refereed and nonrefereed journals, and original research articles, for timeliness, reliability, and applicability before using the information to answer a question.

Textbooks.   Information obtained from textbooks is evaluated from several different perspectives. Note the publication date. Older texts (texts published more than

BOX 9-4

Questions to Ask When Assessing Websites That Provide Health-Related Information

WEBSITE-RELATED QUESTIONS
Who runs the website?
Who pays for the website?
What is the purpose of the website?
Are links current?
Are links appropriate?
Is the website searchable?
Is the date of the last website update posted?
What information does the website collect from users?

AUTHORSHIP-RELATED QUESTIONS
Who controls content?
Are authors identified?
What are the authors' credentials?
Are author credentials related to information provided?
Is there a way to contact authors directly?

INFORMATION-RELATED QUESTIONS
Are opinions separate from fact?
Are facts referenced?
Is the information current?
Is the information relevant?
Is the information balanced?
Is the information peer-reviewed?
Are author-related or site-related financial conflicts identified?

Modified from Ling, CA: Am J Health-Syst Pharm 56:212-214, 1999; Health Summit Working Group: www.hitiweb.mitretek.org/iq; Health on the Net Foundation: www.hon.ch/HONcode/conduct; and National Center for Complementary and Alternative Medicine: www.nccam.nih.gov/health/webre-sources.

4 or 5 years ago) may contain information that was correct at time of publication but is inaccurate based on currently available information. This is especially true for pharmacotherapeutics, pathophysiology, pharmacology, and other medical information. Textbooks also may contain errors; do not accept any information at face value without verification from a second, more recent source.

Note the author of the chapter or book and determine whether the author has the expertise and experience necessary to be an authoritative source of information. Ideally, authors should be practitioners who deal regularly with the issues they are writing about and should be familiar with the literature and state-of-the-art issues relevant to the topic.

Literature Reviews. Literature reviews, also known as *review articles*, are published in refereed and nonrefereed journals, special supplements to journals, and other published formats. Literature reviews provide information somewhat intermediary between original research and textbooks. Literature reviews must be evaluated carefully (Box 9-5).[8-10] As with textbooks, determine the timeliness of the articles by checking the date of publication and assess author expertise.

Assess how the authors selected and evaluated the primary research used as the basis of the review. The purpose of the review should be clearly spelled out in the introduction. Because the conclusions of the review article are based on information obtained from relevant original research, the methodology used to locate the research publications should be identified and outlined. Data obtained from previous review articles should not be used; the authors should locate and assess relevant original data, not another author's interpretation of the data. The criteria for extraction and acceptance of data from the original research should be specific and documented. Determine whether the author's conclusions are supported by the data.

Original Research.   Published research, primarily in the form of clinical trials, is an important source of drug information. Research reports often are cited as proving the usefulness of specific therapeutic agents for new or unapproved indications and as the basis for proving or disproving the association between a drug and a specific adverse drug reaction or interaction. However, original research articles must be evaluated carefully (Box 9-6). The results as stated by the authors cannot be accepted at face value. A thorough and critical appraisal of the research methodology must be completed before the information can be accepted and used for patient care decisions. A single study cannot stand alone in changing clinical practice. Ideally, multiple studies of different patient populations are needed to change clinical practice.[11]

Assess the validity and applicability of the research.[11-13] *Validity* refers to the likelihood that the study results are true. *Applicability* refers to the likelihood that the study results can be useful for clinical decision making. Consider subject characteristics (e.g., age, sex, severity and duration of disease) and decide whether they are similar to those of the patient in question. All studies are flawed; however, study results can be applied to specific patient situations if considered in terms of the strengths and weaknesses of the study.

Clinical appraisal of original research begins with a review of the abstract. Abstracts usually contain enough information to determine whether the study applies to the question at hand and is strong enough to merit further evaluation. Structured abstracts in which the objective, study design, setting, subjects, interventions, main outcome measures, results, and conclusions are clearly identified and

---

BOX 9-5

Questions to Ask When Reviewing Review Articles

1. What are the qualifications of the authors?
2. Was the question clearly stated?
3. Were relevant studies located using a comprehensive search strategy?
4. Were the selection criteria used to select studies explicit and clearly identified?
5. Was each study valid?
6. Were study results combined appropriately?
7. Were the conclusions supported by the combined data?

BOX 9-6

Questions to Ask When Reviewing Original Research

1. What are the qualifications of the investigators?
2. Who funded the study?
3. What are the study's objectives?
4. What is the study design? Is the study design appropriate for the stated objectives?
5. Is a control group used, and if so, is the control group appropriate for the stated objectives?
6. What are the outcome measures? Are the outcome measures appropriate for the stated objectives?
7. Are the data complete? Are all study subjects accounted for? Are any of the data missing?
8. Were the analytical (laboratory) techniques appropriate for the type of samples?
9. Were the statistical analyses appropriate?
10. Are statistically significant results clinically important?
11. Could any uncontrolled factors (e.g., seasonal variations in severity of disease) have influenced the outcome of the study?
12. What is the clinical relevance of the study results?

summarized allow the reader to determine quickly the potential applicability and usefulness of the study.[14]

Look for the study objective. The objective, a statement of the fact, is usually stated in the introductory section of the paper. One of the key components of critical appraisal of original research is to determine whether the authors conducted a study appropriately designed to accomplish the stated objective.

Note the basic study design and determine whether the study design is appropriate for the study objective. For example, interventional studies, commonly used to compare drug regimens, are typically randomized or nonrandomized control trials. These types of studies can be blinded or nonblinded, placebo- or active-controlled, and crossover or parallel in design. It would be difficult to conclude that a new drug is the drug of choice if the study compared the new drug with a placebo rather than the currently accepted drug of choice. Note whether patient adherence to study requirements (e.g., medication, diet, exercise) was assessed and also review the methods used to assess adherence (e.g., pill counts, random blood or urine screens, witnessed drug administration).

Note the study setting and determine whether the setting is appropriate for the study objective. For example, although multicenter trials are difficult to conduct and introduce more chances for study-related errors, multicenter trials are an appropriate study design for rare or unusual disease states or drug treatments.

Note the study participant characteristics and determine whether these characteristics are appropriate for the study objective. Note how study participants were selected (e.g., serial admissions, a random sample from a clinic population, by special invitation), whether the study used normal volunteers or patients, and the patient care setting (e.g., outpatient or inpatient). Consider the median age and range of ages included in the study, the gender distribution of the subjects, and the socioeconomic features of the study population. Explanations of the number of subjects who withdrew and their reasons should be noted; all subjects enrolled in a study should be accounted for in the results.

Assess the study outcome parameters. Note whether the outcome parameters are appropriate for the study objective and whether the parameters used to measure the outcomes are appropriate, comprehensive, and clinically applicable to the study objective.

Review the study results in detail. Look at the data contained in the tables, graphs, and charts in detail to verify the author conclusions and note whether the published conclusions are supported by the data and whether the statistical analyses are appropriate for the study design and types of data. Determine whether the study results, even if statistically significant, are clinically important.

ANSWERING THE QUESTION

Once information is located and analyzed, formulate the answer and convey the answer to the person asking the question. An answer may be as simple as a specific dosage or may require an extensive search for information and the assessment and synthesis of numerous original research articles. In either case the answer must be timely, concise, precise, and appropriate to the background of the person asking the question. The answer should be fully referenced.

Verbal communication of drug information must be clear and fluent. The information should be well organized, with an appropriate emphasis on important details. Convey the answer with confidence and at a level appropriate to the person asking the question. Be prepared to expand on the information according to the needs of the person asking the question.

Written communication of drug information must be well organized, complete, and well written. Use correct sentence and paragraph structure and correct grammar, punctuation, and spelling. Document references in a uniformly accepted format such as that described in the "Uniform Requirements for Manuscripts Submitted to Biomedical Journals."[15]

The written response includes a statement of the question, relevant patient details (e.g., age, disease history, drug history), relevant data from the literature sources, evaluation of the literature cited, summary, conclusions and recommendations, and references. The written response should flow well with smooth transitions between sections. Document the name of the person asking the question and the name of the person answering the question.

File the question, answer, and references for future reference. In some situations (e.g., in drug information centers), a written response to a question is documented in a specific format. In some cases the question and response are written directly in or added to the patient's chart.

DRUG INFORMATION CENTERS

More than 200 pharmacist-operated drug information centers are in operation in the United States.[16] Most of these centers are located in hospitals and run by the hospital's pharmacy department. However, some drug information centers are located in medical libraries, colleges of pharmacy, and poison control centers. Most pharmaceutical companies maintain in-house drug information centers.[17]

The University of Kentucky Drug Information Center was the first drug information center in the United States. It began operation in 1962 as a drug information source, an aid to teaching, an aid in the selection and rational use of drugs, a center for reporting adverse drug reactions, a stimulus for the development of additional drug information centers, and a training site for drug information specialists.[18]

These tasks remain the focus of most drug information centers today. The primary activities of drug information centers include drug information activities; formulary activities; publication of newsletters and other related publications; staff development; investigational drug program activities; drug use review; adverse drug reaction reporting; research; and training of students, pharmacy residents, and drug information specialists.

Drug information specialists are pharmacists who have completed specialized training in drug information, generally in the form of 1-year residency programs in drug information provided by hospitals and other drug information centers. Drug information specialists are skilled in locating and evaluating drug information and in communicating with pharmacists, physicians, other health care providers, and patients.

SELF-ASSESSMENT QUESTIONS

1. Which of the following are important components involved in the provision of drug information?
   a. Determining the primary question
   b. Developing an appropriate search strategy
   c. Assessing available information
   d. All of the above
   e. None of the above
2. A consumer asks whether her new prescription drug is the cause of her insomnia. What type of drug information question is this?
   a. Adverse reaction
   b. Dosing
   c. Drug administration
   d. Indication and therapeutic use
   e. Poisoning and toxicology
3. A colleague asks if ipratropium bromide (Atrovent) is FDA approved for the treatment of asthma. What type of drug information question is this?
   a. Adverse reaction
   b. Dosing
   c. Drug administration
   d. Indication and therapeutic use
   e. Poisoning and toxicology
4. Which one of the following is an example of primary literature?
   a. An original study published in the *New England Journal of Medicine*
   b. A review of a newly marketed drug published in the *Medical Letter*
   c. A drug interaction described in a drug interactions book
5. Which one of the following is an example of secondary literature?
   a. An original study published in the *New England Journal of Medicine*
   b. A review of a newly marketed drug published in the *Medical Letter*
   c. A drug interaction described in a drug interactions book
6. Which one of the following is an example of tertiary literature?
   a. An original study published in the *New England Journal of Medicine*
   b. A review of a newly marketed drug published in the *Medical Letter*
   c. A drug interaction described in a drug interactions book

7. Which of the following is an important consideration when evaluating an original research article?
   a. Appropriateness of the study design
   b. Clinical significance of statistically significant data
   c. Study participant characteristics
   d. All of the above
   e. None of the above

8. Which of the following is an important consideration when evaluating a literature review?
   a. Publication date
   b. Author expertise
   c. How the author selected the primary research articles
   d. All of the above
   e. None of the above

9. Which of the following is the *most* appropriate source of information regarding questions of fact such as usual dosage regimens?
   a. The pharmaceutical company
   b. A colleague
   c. A standard pharmacy textbook
   d. An online search of the published literature
   e. All of the above

10. Which of the following is the *most* appropriate source of information regarding an unapproved indication for a currently marketed drug?
    a. The pharmaceutical company
    b. A colleague
    c. A standard pharmacy textbook
    d. An online search of the published literature
    e. All of the above

References

1. Garfield E: Which medical journals have the greatest impact? *Ann Intern Med* 105:313-320, 1986.
2. Marra CA et al: Drug and poison information resources on the Internet, Part 1: an introduction, *Pharmacotherapy* 16:537-546, 1996.
3. Marra CA et al: Drug and poison information resources on the Internet, Part 2: identification and evaluation, *Pharmacotherapy* 16:806-818, 1996.
4. Ling CA: Guiding patients through the maze of drug information on the Internet, *Am J Health-Syst Pharm* 56:212-214, 1999.
5. Health Summit Working Group: Information quality tool. Available at: www.hitiweb.mitretek.org/iq. Accessed August 9, 2002.
6. Health on the Net Foundation: Code of Conduct (HONcode) for medical and health Websites. Available at: www.hon.ch/HONcode/conduct. Accessed August 9, 2002.
7. National Center for Complementary and Alternative Medicine: 10 things to know about evaluating medical resources on the web. Available at: www.nccam.nih.gov/health/webresources. Accessed August 9, 2002.
8. Morgan PP: Review articles: 1. Looking over the field, *Can Med Assoc J* 134:11, 1986.
9. Morgan PP: Review articles: 2. The literature jungle, *Can Med Assoc J* 134:98-99, 1986.
10. Oxman AD, Guyatt GH: Guidelines for reading literature reviews, *Can Med Assoc J* 138:697-703, 1988.
11. Weintraub M: How to evaluate reports of clinical trials, *P & T* 17:1463-1473, 1990.
12. Fowkes FGR, Fulton PM: Critical appraisal of published research: introductory guidelines, *BMJ* 302:1136-1140, 1991.

13. Gardner MJ, Machin D, Campbell MJ: Use of check lists in assessing the statistical content of medical studies, BMJ 292:810-812, 1986.
14. Haynes RB et al: More informative abstracts revisited, *Ann Intern Med* 113:69-76, 1990.
15. International Committee of Medical Journal Editors: Uniform requirements for manuscripts submitted to biomedical journals, N *Engl* J *Med* 324:424-428, 1991.
16. Beaird SL, Coley RMR, Crea KA: Current status of drug information centers, *Am* J *Hosp Pharm* 49:103-106, 1992.
17. Colvin CL: Understanding the resources and organization of an industry-based drug information service, *Am* J *Hosp Pharm* 47:1989-1990, 1990.
18. Parker PF: The University of Kentucky Drug Information Center, *Am* J *Hosp Pharm* 22:42-47, 1965.

Ethics in Pharmacy and Health Care

10

CHAPTER

Learning Objectives

- Identify the fundamental moral principle on which all ethical behavior is based.
- Describe the commonalities among the pharmacy, medical, and nursing codes of ethics.
- Describe the intent and content of the Patient Care Partnership.
- List actions pharmacists should take to uphold patient confidentiality.
- Identify the two internationally recognized research codes of ethics.
- State the composition and responsibilities of research review boards.
- Identify the required and optional elements of informed consent.
- Describe two ethical implications of accepting gifts from the pharmaceutical industry.
- Differentiate between the purposes of living wills and durable powers of attorney.
- State at least one advantage and disadvantage of living wills and durable powers of attorney.

*E*thics is the science of morality. All ethical behavior is based on the fundamental moral principle of doing good and avoiding evil. Ethical behavior in the profession of pharmacy also means conforming to the rules governing the rights and duties of pharmacists, patients, and other health care professionals.

Health care professionals grapple with many ethical issues (Box 10-1). Some issues, such as the use of animals in drug development, are of interest to health professionals in general but have minimal impact on the daily practice of pharmacy. Other issues, such as confidentiality and withholding or withdrawing specific therapeutic interventions, commonly influence the practice of pharmacy.

This chapter identifies and describes the professional codes of ethics that form the basis of professional ethical behavior and discusses several specific ethical issues, including confidentiality, research ethics, ethics and the promotion of drugs, and the use of advance directives in end-of-life decisions. Additional information regarding biomedical ethical principles is available in the biomedical ethics literature. Detailed specific discussions regarding biomedical ethical issues are published in the medical literature; discussions of specific dispensing-related ethical issues are published in the pharmacy literature.

BOX 10-1

Examples of Health Care–Related Ethical Issues

Abortifacients (e.g., mifepristone)
Assisted reproduction and donation of genetic material
Confidentiality
Euthanasia and assisted suicide
Performance enhancing drugs (e.g., steroids)
Research
    Animal testing
    Biologic research
    Genetic research
    Informed consent
    Investigational drugs
Risk/benefit limitations (e.g., clozapine)
Substance abuse and dependence
Withholding or withdrawing treatment interventions
    Cardiopulmonary resuscitation
    Fluids
    Intubation and ventilation
    Nutrition (tube feedings, total parenteral nutrition)
    Kidney dialysis

PROFESSIONAL CODES OF ETHICS

Most health professions have specific codes of ethics that provide written guidelines regarding ethical behavior. The medical code of ethics, often considered the foundation for ethical behavior in health care, dates to the time of Hippocrates; other codes of ethics are more recent. Most professional codes of ethics are written using broad-based directives that do not provide issue-specific guidelines. This means that the ethical guidelines for most health care professionals are deliberately vague. Therefore to be ethical requires that health professionals apply their professional codes of ethics within a framework of societal moral values. Individual philosophies and beliefs must be considered and respected.

THE HIPPOCRATIC OATH

The Hippocratic oath, attributed to the fifth century BC Greek physician Hippocrates, is considered the basis for modern medical ethical standards.[1] The oath is found in the Hippocratic corpus, a collection of literature containing case reports, descriptions of disease processes, and medical philosophies generally attributed to Hippocrates. Issues addressed in the oath include patient advocacy, patient confidentiality, professional misconduct, and the need to defer to those with more appropriate training and experience (Box 10-2).

THE PHARMACY CODE OF ETHICS

The foundation of ethical pharmacy behavior is the premise that the welfare of humanity is the pharmacist's primary consideration. The declaration that "Every

BOX 10-2

The Hippocratic Oath

I swear by Apollo Physician and Aesculapius and Hygeia and Panacea and all the gods and goddesses, making them my witnesses, that I will fulfill according to my ability and judgment this oath and this covenant: To hold him who has taught me this art as equal to my parents and to live my life in partnership with him, and if he is in need of money to give him a share of mine, and to regard his offspring as equal to my brothers in male lineage and to teach them this art—if they desire to learn it—without fee and covenant; to give a share of precepts and oral instruction and all the other learning to my sons and to the sons of him who has instructed me and to pupils who have signed the covenant and have taken an oath according to medical law, but to no one else. I will apply dietetic measures for the benefit of the sick according to my ability and judgment; I will keep them from harm and injustice. I will neither give a deadly drug to anybody if asked for it, nor will I make a suggestion to this effect. Similarly I will not give to a woman an abortive remedy. In purity and holiness I will guard my life and my art. I will not use the knife, not even on sufferers from stone, but will withdraw in favor of such men as are engaged in this work. Whatever houses I may visit, I will come for the benefit of the sick, remaining free from all intentional injustice, of all mischief and in particular of sexual relations with both female and male persons, be they free or slaves. What I may see or hear in the course of the treatment or even outside of the treatment in regard to the life of men, which on no account one must spread abroad, I will keep to myself holding such things shameful to be spoken about. If I fulfill this oath and do not violate it, may it be granted to me to enjoy life and art, be honored with fame among all men for all time to come; if I transgress it and swear falsely, may the opposite of all this be my lot.

Modified from Temkin O, Temkin CL: *Ancient medicine: selected papers of Ludwig Edelstein*, Baltimore, 1967, Johns Hopkins University

pharmacist shall devote himself carefully and diligently to his task so that the sick and suffering are not neglected and no harm is done to them" was made by a group of pharmacists in 1456.[2] The document containing this statement is considered one of the oldest known ethical commitments made by a group of pharmacists.

The first American pharmacy code of ethics was adopted in 1848 by the Philadelphia College of Pharmacy.[3] This early pharmacy code of ethics states the responsibility of the pharmacist to the patient and recognizes the professional relationship between pharmacists and physicians. The preface to the code includes the following statement[3]:

Pharmacy being a profession which demands knowledge, skill, and integrity on the part of those engaged in it, and being associated with the medical profession in the responsible duties of preserving the public health, and dispensing the useful though often dangerous agents adapted to the cure of disease, its members should be united on some general principle to be observed in their several relations to each other, to the medical profession, and to the public.

Additional components of the code address the need for reasonable remuneration for services and products, the need to distinguish between pure and impure drugs, the need to control the distribution of poisons, and the minimum requirements for education and apprenticeship.

The American Pharmacists Association (APhA), founded in 1852, modeled its first code of ethics after the Philadelphia College of Pharmacy code of ethics. Generally accepted as the professional guidelines for American pharmacists, the APhA code of ethics was revised in 1922, 1952, 1969, 1975, and 1994. The 1994 code of ethics (Box 10-3) differs significantly from earlier codes in that it provides principles based on "moral obligations and virtues" rather than practice-specific guidelines.[4] The 1994 code for the first time defines the pharmacist-patient relationship as a covenant, implying moral obligations such as compassion, caring, honesty, and integrity.[5]

The duty to accept the profession's ethical principles is further emphasized by the oath of the pharmacist[6] (Box 10-4). The oath, traditionally taken at the time of graduation from pharmacy school, states that the primary concern of the pharmacist is the welfare of humanity and relief of human suffering and that the pharmacist is expected to maintain the highest standards of moral and ethical conduct.

PHYSICIAN AND NURSING CODES OF ETHICS

The American Medical Association established the first American medical code of ethics in 1847. The code was first revised in 1906 after several decades of discussion and turmoil.[7] The current code, revised in 2001, describes the responsibilities of the physician to patients, society, other health care professionals, and self and establishes specific standards of conduct[8] (Box 10-5). The Florence Nightingale Pledge was written in 1893 by a group of nurses in Detroit.[9] The Code of Ethics for Nurses (Box 10-6) describes the goals, values, and obligations of the nursing profession.

BOX 10-3

The Code of Ethics for Pharmacists

PREAMBLE

Pharmacists are health professionals who assist individuals in making the best use of medications. This Code, prepared and supported by pharmacists, is intended to state publicly the principles that form the fundamental basis of the roles and responsibilities of pharmacists. These principles, based on moral obligations and virtues, are established to guide pharmacists in relationships with patients, health professionals, and society.

PRINCIPLES

    I. A pharmacist respects the covenantal relationship between the patient and pharmacist.

    II. A pharmacist promotes the good of every patient in a caring, compassionate, and confidential manner.

    III. A pharmacist respects the autonomy and dignity of each patient.

    IV. A pharmacist acts with honesty and integrity in professional relationships.

    V. A pharmacist maintains professional competence.

    VI. A pharmacist respects the values and abilities of colleagues and other health professionals.

    VII. A pharmacist serves individual, community, and societal needs.

    VIII. A pharmacist seeks justice in the distribution of health resources.

From *Code of ethics for pharmacists*, Washington, DC, 1995, American Pharmaceutical Association.

BOX 10-4

Oath of a Pharmacist

At this time, I vow to devote my professional life to the service of all humankind through the profession of pharmacy. I will consider the welfare of humanity and relief of human suffering my primary concerns. I will apply my knowledge, experience, and skills to the best of my ability to assure optimal drug therapy outcomes for the patients I serve. I will keep abreast of developments and maintain professional competency in my profession of pharmacy. I will maintain the highest principles of moral, ethical, and legal conduct. I will embrace and advocate change in the profession of pharmacy that improves patient care. I take these vows voluntarily with the full realization of the responsibility with which I am entrusted by the public.

From *Oath of a pharmacist*, Alexandria, VA, 1995, American Association of Colleges of Pharmacy.

BOX 10-5

American Medical Association Principles of Medical Ethics

PREAMBLE
The medical profession has long subscribed to a body of ethical statements developed primarily for the benefit of the patient. As a member of this profession, a physician must recognize responsibility to patients first and foremost, as well as to society, to other health professionals, and to self. The following Principles adopted by the American Medical Association are not laws, but standards of conduct which define the essentials of honorable behavior for the physician.

  I. A physician shall be dedicated to providing competent medical service with compassion and respect for human dignity and rights.

  II. A physician shall uphold the standards of professionalism, be honest in all professional interactions, and strive to report physicians deficient in character or competence, or engaging in fraud or deception, to appropriate entities.

  III. A physician shall respect the law and also recognize a responsibility to seek changes in those requirements which are contrary to the best interests of the patient.

  IV. A physician shall respect the rights of patients, of colleagues, and of other health professionals, and shall safeguard patient confidences within the constraints of the law.

  V. A physician shall continue to study, apply and advance scientific knowledge, maintain a commitment to medical education, make relevant information available to patients, colleagues, and the public, obtain consultation, and use the talents of other health professionals when indicated.

  VI. A physician shall, in the provision of appropriate patient care, except in emergencies, be free to chose whom to serve, with whom to associate, and the environment in which to provide medical services.

  VII. A physician shall recognize a responsibility to participate in activities contributing to the improvement of the community and the betterment of public health.

  VIII. A physician shall, while caring for a patient, regard responsibility to the patient as paramount.

  IX. A physician shall support access to medical care for all people.

From Principles of Medical Ethics. Available at: www.ama-asn.org/ama/pub/category. Accessed August 8, 2002.

Code of Ethics for Nurses

Provision 1. The nurse, in all professional relationships, practices with compassion and respect for the inherent dignity, worth, and uniqueness of every individual, unrestricted by considerations of social or economic status, personal attributes, or the nature of health problems.

Provision 2. The nurse's primary commitment is to the patient, whether an individual, family, group, or community.

Provision 3. The nurse promotes, advocates for, and strives to protect the health, safety, and rights of the patient.

Provision 4. The nurse is responsible and accountable for individual nursing practice and determines the appropriate delegation of tasks consistent with the nurse's obligation to provide optimum patient care.

Provision 5. The nurse owes the same duties to self as to others, including the responsibility to preserve integrity and safety, to maintain competence, and to continue personal and professional growth.

Provision 6. The nurse participates in establishing, maintaining, and improving health care environments and conditions of employment conducive to the provision of quality health care and consistent with the values of the profession, through individual and collective action.

Provision 7. The nurse participates in the advancement of the profession through contributions to practice, education, administration, and knowledge development.

Provision 8. The nurse collaborates with other health professionals and the public in promoting community, national, and international efforts to meet health needs.

Provision 9. The profession of nursing, as represented by associations and their members, is responsible for articulating nursing values, for maintaining the integrity of the profession and its practice, and for shaping social policy.

From American Nurses Association Code of Ethics for Nurses.[10]

PATIENT RIGHTS

Patients are autonomous and have the ethical and legal right to make decisions regarding their health care. However, patients may lose their sense of autonomy when hospitalized and may not understand their rights as individuals. The Patient Care Partnership: Understanding Expectations, Rights, and Responsibilities (Box 10-7)[11] describes institutional and patient responsibilities.

ETHICAL ISSUES

Guidelines for ethical issues such as patient confidentiality and clinical research are well established and apply to all health care professionals. Some ethical issues such as the relationship between the pharmaceutical industry and health care professionals are relatively new. Other issues such as the role of the pharmacist in decisions regarding discontinuation of medical treatment are just being identified; ethical guidelines may take years to develop.

BOX 10-7

The Patient Care Partnership: Understanding Expectations, Rights, and Responsibilities

When you need hospital care, your doctor and the nurses and other professionals at our hospital are committed to working with you and your family to meet your health care needs. Our dedicated doctors and staff serve the community in all its ethnic, religious, and economic diversity. Our goal is for you and your family to have the same care and attention we would want for our families and ourselves.

The sections below explain some of the basics about how you can expect to be treated during your hospital stay. They also cover what we will need from you to care for you better. If you have questions at any time, please ask them. Unasked or unanswered questions can add to the stress of being in the hospital. Your comfort and confidence in your care are very important to us.

WHAT TO EXPECT DURING YOUR HOSPITAL STAY

High quality care. Our first priority is to provide you the care you need, when you need it, with skill, compassion, and respect. Tell your caregivers if you have concerns about your care or if you have pain. You have the right to know the identity of doctors, nurses, and others involved in your care, as well as when they are students, residents, or other trainees.

A clean and safe environment. Our hospital works hard to keep you safe. We use special policies and procedures to avoid mistakes in your care and keep you free from abuse or neglect. If anything unexpected and significant happens during your hospital stay, you will be told what happened and any resulting changes in your care will be discussed with you.

Involvement in your care. You and your doctor often make decisions about your care before you go to the hospital. Other times, especially in emergencies, those decisions are made during your hospital stay. When they take place, making decisions should include:

Discussing your medical condition and information about medically appropriate treatment choices. To make informed decisions with your doctor, you need to understand several things:

- The benefits and risks of each treatment.
- Whether it is experimental or part of a research study.
- What you can reasonably expect from your treatment and any long-term effects it might have on your quality of life.
- What you and your family will need to do after you leave the hospital.
- The financial consequences of using uncovered services or out-of-network providers.

Please tell your caregivers if you need more information about treatment choices.

Discussing your treatment plan. When you enter the hospital, you sign a general consent to treatment. In some cases, such as surgery or experimental treatment, you may be asked to confirm in writing that you understand what is planned and agree to it. This process protects your right to consent to or refuse a treatment. Your doctor will explain the medical consequences of refusing recommended treatment. It also protects your right to decide if you want to participate in a research study.

Getting information from you. Your caregivers need complete and correct information about your health and coverage so that they can make good decisions about your care. That includes:

- Past illnesses, surgeries, or hospital stays.
- Past allergic reactions.

BOX 10-7

The Patient Care Partnership: Understanding Expectations, Rights, and Responsibilities—cont'd

- Any medicines or diet supplements (such as vitamins and herbs) that you are taking.
- Any network or admission requirements under your health plan.

Understanding your health care goals and values. You may have health care goals and values or spiritual beliefs that are important to your well-being. They will be taken into account as much as possible throughout your hospital stay. Make sure your doctor, your family, and your care team know your wishes.

Understanding who should make decisions when you cannot. If you have signed a health care power of attorney stating who should speak for you if you become unable to make health care decisions for yourself, or a "living will" or "advance directive" that states your wishes about end-of-life care, give copies to your doctor, your family and your care team. If you or your family need help making difficult decisions, counselors, chaplains and others are available to help.

Protection of your privacy. We respect the confidentiality of your relationship with your doctor and other caregivers, and the sensitive information about your health and health care that are part of that relationship. State and federal laws and hospital operating policies protect the privacy of your medical information. You will receive a Notice of Privacy Practices that describes the ways that we use, disclose, and safeguard patient information and that explains how you can obtain a copy of information from our records about your care.

Help preparing you and your family for when you leave the hospital. Your doctor works with hospital staff and professionals in your community. You and your family also play an important role. The success of your treatment often depends on your efforts to follow medication, diet, and therapy plans. Your family may need to help care for you at home.

You can expect us to help you identify sources of follow-up care and to let you know if your hospital has a financial interest in any referrals. As long as you agree we can share information about your care with them, we will coordinate our activities with your caregivers outside the hospital. You can also expect to receive information and, where possible, training about the self-care you will need when you go home.

Help with your bill and filing insurance claims. Our staff will file claims for you with health care insurers or other programs such as Medicare and Medicaid. They will also help your doctor with needed documentation. Hospital bills and insurance coverage are often confusing. If you have questions about your bill, contact our business office. If you need help understanding your insurance coverage or health plan, start with your insurance company or health benefits manager. If you do not have health coverage, we will try to help you and your family find financial help or make other arrangements. We need your help with collecting needed information and other requirements to obtain coverage or assistance.

While you are here, you will receive more detailed notices about some of the rights you have as a hospital patient and how to exercise them. We are always interested in improving. If you have questions, comments, or concerns, please contact _____.

CONFIDENTIALITY

Confidentiality of patient information is a common ethical issue that all health care professionals address daily. The moral concept of confidentiality is present in many religious philosophies and was initially documented for the medical profession in the Hippocratic oath. The Hippocratic oath states, "What I may see or hear in the course of treatment or even outside of the treatment in regard to the life of men, which on no account one must spread abroad, I will keep to myself holding such things shameful to be spoken about."[1] Most health care professions provide guidelines regarding confidentiality of patient information.

Confidentiality of patient information is maintained not only out of respect for the basic moral right of the patient to privacy but also to encourage patients to entrust pharmacists with the details of their illnesses and uses of medications. An environment that ensures patients that information discussed with the pharmacist will be used only by those involved in their care must be created. Few patients would be willing to admit to noncompliance with prescribed medication regimens or would discuss drug abuse if they thought the information would become public.

To uphold patient confidentiality, restrict access to written and computerized patient records, including medication histories and patient monitoring records. Do not discuss specific patient cases in public areas. Discussions with patients and discussions about specific patient cases should be held in private settings, such as consultation rooms, conference rooms, or other private areas. Do not discuss patient case information in public areas such as hallways, elevators, and cafeterias.

RESEARCH ETHICS

Research is an important activity for many pharmacists. Pharmacists often serve as principal investigators or coinvestigators. Other research-related responsibilities include protocol development; grantsmanship; and administrative responsibilities, such as obtaining institutional approval for research, enrolling subjects, obtaining informed consent, dispensing, ensuring inventory control, collecting data, analyzing data, and reporting results.

The need for universally accepted ethical standards evolved as types and numbers of research protocols increased. Historical misconduct added to the need for universal ethical standards. For example, research in the midtwentieth century often was conducted on prisoners, mentally incompetent persons, and patients in insane asylums; little consideration was given to the ethics of such research or the rights of the participants, who were often viewed as less than human.[12] Nazis' abuse of prisoners during World War II led to the development of the Nuremberg code, an internationally recognized research code of ethics (Box 10-8).[13] The World Medical Association Declaration of Helsinki, derived from the Nuremberg Code, is a widely accepted international code of research ethics (Box 10-9).[14]

In addition to complying with internationally accepted research codes of ethics, pharmacists must comply with federal regulations regarding the rights of research subjects. The federal regulations consist of the Department of Health and Human Services (DHHS) Code of Federal Regulations (CFR) Title 45A, part 46 and Title 21 of the Food and Drug Administration.[15] These regulations describe the composition and function of institutional review boards (IRBs), define the elements of informed consent, and provide the guidelines for documentation of informed consent.

The purpose of an IRB, also known as a *human research review board (HRRB)* or *human investigation committee (HIC)*, is to safeguard the rights and welfare of human research subjects. Investigators must submit all research protocols to the board and

BOX 10-8

The Nuremberg Code

The great weight of evidence before us is to the effect that certain types of medical experiments on human beings, when kept within reasonably well-defined bounds, conform to the ethics of the medical profession generally. The protagonists of the practice of human experimentation justify their views on the basis that such experiments yield results for the good of society that are unprocurable by other methods or means of study. All agree, however that certain basic principles must be observed in order to satisfy moral, ethical, and legal concepts.

1. The voluntary consent of the human subject is absolutely essential.
2. The experiment should be such as to yield fruitful results for the good of society, unprocurable by other methods or means of study, and not random and unnecessary in nature.
3. The experiment should be so designed and based on the results of animal experimentation and a knowledge of the natural history of the disease or other problem under study that the anticipated results will justify the performance of the experiment.
4. The experiment should be so conducted as to avoid all unnecessary physical and mental suffering and injury.
5. No experiment should be conducted where there is an *a priori* reason to believe that death or disabling injury will occur; except, perhaps, in those experiments where the experimental physicians also serve as subjects.
6. The degree of risk to be taken should never exceed that determined by the humanitarian importance of the problem to be solved by the experiment.
7. Proper preparations should be made and adequate facilities provided to protect the experimental subject against even remote possibilities of injury, disability, or death.
8. The experiment should be conducted only by scientifically qualified persons. The highest degree of skill and care should be required through all stages of the experiment of those who conduct or engage in the experiment.
9. During the course of the experiment the human subject should be at liberty to bring the experiment to an end if he has reached the physical or mental state where continuation of the experiment seems to him to be impossible.
10. During the course of the experiment the scientist in charge must be prepared to terminate the experiment at any stage, if he has probably [sic] cause to believe, in the exercise of the good faith, superior skill and careful judgment required of him that a continuation of the experiment is likely to result in injury, disability, or death to the experimental subject.

From *Trials of war criminals before the Nuremberg military tribunals under control council law* 10:181-182, October 1946-April 1949.

obtain approval before performing the research. Each institution in which human research is conducted must have this type of board. Noninstitution human research review boards are available for researchers engaged in clinical research outside specific institutions.[16]

The composition of research review boards is defined by law. Each board must be composed of at least five members with varying backgrounds capable of reviewing

BOX 10-9

The Declaration of Helsinski

INTRODUCTION

The World Medical Association has developed the Declaration of Helsinski as a statement of ethical principles to provide guidance to physicians and other participants in medical research involving human subjects. Medical research involving human subjects includes research on identifiable human material or identifiable data.

It is the duty of the physician to promote and safeguard the health of the people. The physician's knowledge and conscience are dedicated to the fulfillment of this duty.

The Declaration of Geneva of the World Medical Association binds the physician with the words, "The health of my patient will be my first consideration," and the International Code of Medical Ethics declares that, "A physician shall act only in the patient's interest when providing medical care which might have the effect of weakening the physical and mental condition of the patient."

Medical progress is based on research which ultimately must rest in part on experimentation involving human subjects. In medical research on human subjects, considerations related to the well-being of the human subject should take precedence over the interests of science and society.

The primary purpose of medical research involving human subjects is to improve prophylactic, diagnostic and therapeutic procedures and the understanding of the aetiology and pathogenesis of disease. Even the best proven prophylactic, diagnostic, and therapeutic methods must continuously be challenged through research for their effectiveness, efficiency, accessibility and quality.

In current medical practice and in medical research, most prophylactic, diagnostic and therapeutic procedures involve risks and burdens.

Medical research is subject to ethical standards that promote respect for all human beings and protect their health and rights. Some research populations are vulnerable and need special protection. The particular needs of the economically and medically disadvantaged must be recognized. Special attention is also required for those who cannot give or refuse consent for themselves, for those who will not benefit personally from the research and for those for whom the research is combined with care.

Research investigators should be aware of the ethical, legal and regulatory requirements for research on human subjects in their own countries as well as applicable international requirements. No national ethical, legal or regulatory requirement should be allowed to reduce or eliminate any of the protections for human subjects set forth in this Declaration.

BASIC PRINCIPLES FOR ALL MEDICAL RESEARCH

It is the duty of the physician in medical research to protect the life, health, privacy, and dignity of the human subject.

Medical research involving human subjects must conform to generally accepted scientific principles, be based on a thorough knowledge of the scientific literature, other relevant sources of information, and on adequate laboratory and, where appropriate, animal experimentation.

Appropriate caution must be exercised in the conduct of research which may affect the environment, and the welfare of animals used for research must be respected.

The design and performance of each experimental procedure involving human subjects should be clearly formulated in an experimental protocol. This protocol should be

BOX 10-9

The Declaration of Helsinski—cont'd

submitted for consideration, comment, guidance, and where appropriate, approval to a specially appointed ethical review committee, which must be independent of the investigator, the sponsor or any other kind of undue influence. This independent committee should be in conformity with the laws and regulations of the country in which the research experiment is performed. The committee has the right to monitor ongoing trials. The researcher has the obligation to provide monitoring information to the committee, especially any serious adverse events. The researcher should also submit to the committee, for review, information regarding funding, sponsors, institutional affiliations, other potential conflicts of interest and incentives for subjects.

The research protocol should always contain a statement of the ethical considerations involved and should indicate that there is compliance with the principles enunciated in this Declaration.

Medical research involving human subjects should be conducted only by scientifically qualified persons and under the supervision of a clinically competent medical person. The responsibility for the human subject must always rest with a medically qualified person and never rest on the subject of the research, even though the subject has given consent.

Every medical research project involving human subjects should be preceded by careful assessment of predictable risks and burdens in comparison with foreseeable benefits to the subject or to others. This does not preclude the participation of healthy volunteers in medical research. The design of all studies should be publicly available.

Physicians should abstain from engaging in research projects involving human subjects unless they are confident that the risks involved have been adequately assessed and can be satisfactorily managed. Physicians should cease any investigation if the risks are found to outweigh the potential benefits or if there is conclusive proof of positive and beneficial results.

Medical research involving human subjects should only be conducted if the importance of the objective outweighs the inherent risks and burdens to the subject. This is especially important when the human subjects are healthy volunteers.

Medical research is only justified if there is a reasonable likelihood that the populations in which the research is carried out stand to benefit from the results of the research.

The subjects must be volunteers and informed participants in the research project.

The right of research subjects to safeguard their integrity must always be respected. Every precaution should be taken to respect the privacy of the subject, the confidentiality of the patient's information and to minimize the impact of the study on the subject's physical and mental integrity and on the personality of the subject.

In any research on human beings, each potential subject must be adequately informed of the aims, methods, sources of funding, any possible conflicts of interest, institutional affiliations of the researcher, the anticipated benefits and potential risks of the study and the discomfort it may entail. The subjects should be informed of the right to abstain from participation in the study or to withdraw consent to participate at any time without reprisal. After ensuring that the subject has understood the information, the physician should then obtain the subject's freely-given informed consent, preferably in writing. If the consent cannot be obtained in writing, the non-written consent must be formally documented and witnessed.

When obtaining informed consent for the research project the physician should be particularly cautious if the subject is in a dependent relationship with the physician or may

Continued

BOX 10-9

The Declaration of Helsinski—cont'd

consent under duress. In that case the informed consent should be obtained by a well-informed physician who is not engaged in the investigation and who is completely independent of the relationship.

For a research subject who is legally incompetent, physically or mentally incapable of giving consent or is a legally incompetent minor, the investigator must obtain informed consent from the legally authorized representative in accordance with applicable law. These groups should not be included in research unless the research is necessary to promote the health of the population represented and this research cannot instead be performed on legally competent persons.

When a subject deemed legally incompetent, such as a minor child, is able to give assent to decisions about participation in research, the investigator must obtain that assent in addition to the consent of the legally authorized representative.

Research on individuals from whom it is not possible to obtain consent, including proxy or advance consent, should be done only if the physical/mental condition that prevents obtaining informed consent is a necessary characteristic of the research population. The specific reasons for involving research subjects with a condition that renders them unable to give informed consent should be stated in the experimental protocol for consideration and approval of the review committee. The protocol should state that consent to remain in the research should be obtained as soon as possible from the individual or a legally authorized surrogate.

Both authors and publishers have ethical obligations. In publication of the results of research, the investigators are obliged to preserve the accuracy of the results. Negative as well as positive results should be published or otherwise publicly available. Sources of funding, institutional affiliations and any possible conflicts of interests should be declared in the publication. Reports of experimentation not in accordance with the principles laid down in the Declaration should not be accepted for publication.

ADDITIONAL PRINCIPLES FOR MEDICAL RESEARCH COMBINED WITH MEDICAL CARE

The physician may combine medical research with medical care, only to the extent that the research is justified by its potential prophylactic, diagnostic or therapeutic value. When medical research is combined with medical care, additional standards apply to protect the patients who are research subjects.

The benefits, risks, burdens and effectiveness of a new method should be tested against those of the best current prophylactic, diagnostic, and therapeutic methods. This does not exclude the use of placebo, or no treatment, in studies where no proven prophylactic, diagnostic or therapeutic method exists.[1]

At the conclusion of the study, every patient entered into the study should be assured of access to the best proven prophylactic, diagnostic, and therapeutic methods identified by the study.

The physician should fully inform the patient which aspects of the care are related to the research. The refusal of a patient to participate in a study must never interfere with the patient-physician relationship.

In the treatment of a patient, where proven prophylactic, diagnostic and therapeutic methods do not exist or have been ineffective, the physician, with informed consent from

BOX 10-9

The Declaration of Helsinski—cont'd

the patient, must be free to use unproven or new prophylactic, diagnostic, and therapeutic measures, if in the physician's judgment it offers hope of saving life, re-establishing health, or alleviating suffering. Where possible, these measures should be made the object of research, designed to evaluate their safety and efficacy. In all cases, new information should be recorded and, where appropriate, published. The other relevant guidelines of this Declaration should be followed.

[1]The WMA hereby reaffirms its position that extreme care must be taken in making use of a placebo-controlled trial and that in general this methodology should only be used in the absence of existing proven therapy. However, a placebo-controlled trial may be ethically acceptable, even if proven therapy is available, under the following circumstances: Where for compelling and scientifically sound method-ological reasons its use is necessary to determine the efficacy or safety of a prophylactic, diagnostic or therapeutic method; or Where a prophylactic, diagnostic or therapeutic method is being investigated for a minor condition and the patients who receive placebo will not be subject to any additional risk or seri-ous or irreversible harm.

All other provisions of the Declaration of Helsinki must be adhered to, especially the need for appro-priate ethical and scientific review.

Adopted by the 18th WMA General Assembly, Helsinki, Finland, June 1964 and amended by the
29th WMA General Assembly, Tokyo, Japan, October 1975
35th WMA General Assembly, Venice, Italy, October 1983
41st WMA General Assembly, Hong Kong, September 1989
48th WMA General Assembly, Somerset West, Republic of South Africa, October 1996 and the
52nd WMA General Assembly, Edinburgh, Scotland, October 2000
The WMA General Assembly added a Note of Clarification on paragraph 29, Washington 2002.
Reprinted with permission of the World Medical Association.

the types of research submitted to the board. Board membership also must be diverse. The board cannot be composed of all men, all women, or members of just one profession. At least one board member must be a nonscientist such as a lawyer, ethicist, or member of the clergy, and at least one member must not otherwise be associated with the institution sponsoring the board.

Approval of research proposals is based on decisions regarding the relative risk to subjects, subject identification and selection, consent procedures and documenta-tion, and how subject confidentiality is maintained. Research subjects must be informed to maintain the ethical principle of self-determination. Although the pri-mary purpose of the board is to protect the rights of subjects, the board may com-ment on study design issues and the scientific merit of proposals.

A primary focus of the board is the content of the consent form and how consent is obtained and documented. Written informed consent is required for most human research; consent for some relatively low-risk protocols may be obtained verbally. For consent to be valid, it must be voluntary. The written information must be in lay terms. Exculpatory language cannot be used, and subjects must be considered legally competent. Federal regulations define required and additional elements of informed consent. Consent forms must contain specific elements; other elements are optional (Box 10-10).

BOX 10-10

Elements of Informed Consent[15]

BASIC ELEMENTS OF INFORMED CONSENT
1. A statement that the study involves research and an explanation of the purposes of the research
2. The expected duration of the subject's participation in the study, a description of the procedures to be followed, and identification of experimental procedures
3. A description of reasonably foreseeable risks or discomforts to the subject
4. A statement on the availability of medical treatments and compensation in case the subject is injured by participation in the study
5. A description of benefits to the subjects or others that may reasonably be expected from the research
6. A disclosure of alternatives to participating in the research study
7. A statement describing the extent to which confidentiality will be maintained and noting that the Food and Drug Administration may see the subject's record
8. An explanation of whom to contact for answers to questions about the research and subject's rights and whom to contact in the event a research-related injury occurs
9. A noncoercive disclaimer that participation is voluntary, refusal to participate involves no penalty or loss of benefits, and the subject may discontinue participation at any time without penalty or loss of benefits

OPTIONAL ELEMENTS
1. A statement that the treatment or procedure may involve risks to the subject (or embryo or fetus, if the subject is or becomes pregnant) which are currently unforeseeable
2. Circumstances under which the subject's participation may be terminated by the investigator without the subject's consent
3. Additional costs to the subject from participating in the research
4. Consequences of a subject's decision to withdraw from the research and procedures for orderly termination of participation by the subject
5. A statement that significant new findings during the course of research that may relate to the subject's willingness to continue to participate will be given to the subject
6. The approximate number of subjects in the study

21CFR50.25. Revised as of April 1, 2002.

ETHICS AND THE PROMOTION OF PRESCRIPTION DRUGS

Health care professionals have begun to question the ethics of accepting gifts from drug companies.[17-19] Gifts range from low-cost items such as pens, notepads, clothing, textbooks, and meals to high-cost gifts such as all-expense-paid trips to luxury resorts and cash gifts. Pharmacists attending national pharmacy association meetings often attend industry-sponsored continuing education presentations, receptions, and parties and collect numerous gifts from industry-sponsored exhibits.

The ethical issues are complex and evolve from the unique relationship between the pharmaceutical industry and health care professionals. Unlike other types of advertising, pharmaceutical advertising targets health care professionals, who influence drug selection, and not patients, the ultimate consumers of the products. Ethical implications arise from accepting these gifts, no matter the monetary value of the gift.

The ethical implications of accepting gifts from the pharmaceutical industry involve issues of justness and obligations.[19] The cost of pharmaceutical gifts and other forms of advertising is included in the price of medications. Therefore some argue that spending patients' money without their knowledge or consent and without direct benefit is unjust. Gift giving also implies obligations on the part of the recipient. The obligations may be subtle, but even the appearance of an obligation may alter society's trust in the profession.

Guidelines regarding the relationships of health care professionals with the pharmaceutical industry are evolving. Although most of the discussions have targeted physicians, the ethical issues and therefore the guidelines are applicable to other health care professionals. The American Society of Health-System Pharmacists (ASHP) board of directors approved and published the ASHP guidelines on pharmacists' relationships with industry in 1992.[20] The guidelines address the issues of gifts and hospitality, continuing education, consultants and advisory arrangements, clinical research, and disclosure of information.

Guidelines regarding the relationships of pharmaceutical industry and health professionals also are evolving. The Pharmaceutical Research and Manufacturers of America (PhRMA) adopted a voluntary Code on Interactions with Healthcare Professional in 2002.[21] The code addresses the interactions of pharmaceutical and biotechnology companies with health care professionals, including industry-sponsored informational presentations and educational meetings and the arrangement with consultants.

ADVANCE DIRECTIVES

Advance directives are written legal documents that give a patient the ability to influence future treatment decisions should the patient lose the ability to make decisions. Advance directives are the focus of the Patient Self-Determination Act (PSDA), a law that went into effect on December 1, 1991.[22] The intent of the PSDA is to promote the knowledge and use of advance directives. The law, which applies to all health care institutions (hospitals, nursing facilities, hospices, home care programs, and health maintenance organizations) that receive Medicare or Medicaid, requires institutions to give all individuals receiving medical care written information about their rights under state law to make decisions about their care, including the right to accept or refuse medical or surgical care. Individuals also must be given information about their rights to formulate advance directives. Institutions must prepare policies consistent with state law, document in each individual's medical record whether the individual has executed an advance directive, and develop public education programs.

The two main types of advance directives are living wills (Box 10-11) and durable powers of attorney (Box 10-12); some hybrid documents combine elements of each document. A living will provides direction regarding specific medical treatments the person does or does not want at the end of life and can serve as a general reference for decision making. The advantage of living wills is that individuals can identify specific interventions, such as surgery, dialysis, chest compression, and intubation and mechanical ventilation, they do not want. Living wills are especially useful for patients with chronic illnesses. However, living wills require that individuals predict future acceptable and unacceptable medical interventions, often without an

BOX 10-11

Example of a Living Will

To my Doctor:

While I have been at _____, I have discussed my wishes concerning my medical treatment in the event that I become extremely ill. I did this in the hope that if I made my wishes known beforehand, it would be easier for my doctors to know my preferences at a time when I am unable to express them.

If I become critically ill:

I want to be hospitalized.
I want to go into intensive care.
I want to have my heart revived if my heart stops.
I want to have surgery.
I want to be put on a breathing machine.

If I become terminally ill:

I want to be hospitalized.
I want my family members to decide whether I shall go into intensive care after they talk with my doctor.
I want my doctor to decide whether to revive me if my heart stops.
I want my family members to decide whether I shall have surgery after they talk with my doctor.
I want my family members to decide whether I shall be put on a breathing machine after they talk with my doctor.

If I am in an irreversible coma:

I want to be hospitalized.
I want my family members to decide whether I shall go into intensive care after they talk with my doctor.

I want my doctor to decide whether to revive me if my heart stops.
I want my family members to decide whether I shall have surgery after they talk with my doctor.
I do not want to be put on a breathing machine.
I want my family members to decide whether I shall be fed through a tube after they talk with my doctor.

If I am unable to make decisions for myself, I would like the following person to make necessary decisions on my behalf:

1. Name (relationship)
   Address

   Phone: (home)
          (work)

If you cannot reach _____, I would like the following person to make the necessary decisions on my behalf:
2. Name (relationship)
   Address

   Phone: (home)
          (work)

There will be a time when I want my doctor to stop keeping me alive.

I have provided this information in the hope that it will be easier to respect my wishes about my medical care at a time when I am unable to express them.

Patient name	_____	_____	_____
	(printed)	(signature)	(date)
Witness name	_____	_____	_____
	(printed)	(signature)	(date)

From Danis M et al: A prospective study of advance directives for life-sustaining care, N Engl J Med 324:8882, 1991.

BOX 10-12

Example of a Durable Power of Attorney

I, _____, residing at
(principal—print your name)

_____
(street)   (city or town)   (state)

appoint as my Health Care Agent _____
(name of person you choose as agent)

of _____
(street)   (city or town)   (state)   (phone)

Optional: If my agent is unwilling or unable to serve, then I appoint as my alternate

_____
(name of person you choose as alternate)

of _____
(street)   (city or town)   (state)   (phone)

My agent shall have the authority to make all health care decisions for me, subject to any limitations I state below, if I am unable to make decisions myself. My agent's authority becomes effective if my attending physician determines in writing that I lack the capacity to make or to communicate health care decisions. My agent is then to have the same authority to make health care decisions as I would if I had the capacity to make them, *except* (here list the limitations, *if any,* you wish to place on your agent's authority):

I direct my agent to make decisions on the basis of my agent's assessment of my personal wishes. If my personal wishes are unknown, my agent is to make decisions on the basis of my agent's assessment of my best interests. Photocopies of this Health Care Proxy shall have the same force and effect as the original.

Signed _____

Complete only if principal is physically unable to sign: I have signed the principal's name above at his or her direction in the presence of the principal and two witnesses.

_____
(name)

_____
(street)

_____
(city or town)   (state)

Witness Statement

We, the undersigned, each witnessed the signing of this Health Care Proxy by the principal or at the direction of the principal and state that the principal appears to be at least 18 years of age, of sound mind, and under no constraint or undue influence. Neither of us is named as the health care agent or alternate in this document.

Continued

BOX 10-12

Example of a Durable Power of Attorney—cont'd

In our presence this _____ day of _____ 20_____.

Witness 1 _____   Witness 2 _____
                    (signature)   (signature)

Name (print) _____   Name (print) _____

Address _____   Address _____

_____   _____

From Annas GJ: The health care proxy and the living will, N Engl J Med 324:1210-1213, 1991.

accurate or complete understanding of all available options or the implications of each option. Living wills do not appoint an alternate decision maker and often must be interpreted when tough decisions have to be made regarding end-of-life treatment decisions. Written durable powers of attorney appoint an alternate decision maker (the proxy) who is legally empowered to make decisions regarding the care of the patient. A durable power of attorney is activated whenever the patient is incapacitated. The advantage of the durable power of attorney is that an individual can identify a person to engage in future discussions regarding specific clinical situations. However, the durable power of attorney does not by itself tell the proxy the decisions to make on the patient's behalf. The scope of proxy responsibilities varies by state statute but generally empowers the proxy to admit the person to an acute or chronic care facility and arrange for and consent to medical and surgical treatment.

One of the most common problems associated with advance directives is that the document may not be available when decisions have to be made. The document may be locked in a safe deposit box, filed in a lawyer's office, or held by distant offspring. Another problem is that the document may be out of date and not accurately reflect the patient's desires as the patient faces the realities of end-of-life illnesses and gains experience with available technology and other interventions. Pharmacists should be aware of the presence of advance directives and ensure that therapeutic decisions are made in accordance with the patient's wishes.

WITHHOLDING AND WITHDRAWING MEDICAL INTERVENTIONS

Withholding of life support and *withdrawal of life support* refer to decisions to withhold or withdraw medical interventions with the expectation that the patient will die from the change in support.[25] Technologic and pharmaceutical advances provide health care professionals with effective tools for prolonging life. At issue, however, are the quality of life and the right of patients to make their own decisions. Competent patients or alternate decision makers have the right to choose. Health care professionals have the ethical responsibility to inform patients and alternate decision makers of choices and honor their decisions. Although the responsibility for withholding or withdrawing life support rests with the patient or proxy and the patient's physician, broad consensus is sought among all health professionals involved in the care of the patient. Every effort is made to honor the patient's wishes regarding these difficult decisions.

SELF-ASSESSMENT QUESTIONS

1. Which of the following is the fundamental moral principle on which all ethical behavior is based?
   a. Do good and avoid evil.
   b. Do what is best for society as a whole.
   c. Obey all federal laws.
   d. Maintain patient confidentiality.
   e. Obey all state laws.

2. What do the pharmacy, nursing, and medical codes of ethics have in common?
   a. Hippocrates wrote all three codes.
   b. All contain issue-specific guidelines.
   c. All are based on the Declaration of Helsinki.
   d. All were written in the sixth century BC.
   e. All provide broad-based directives.

3. The Patient Care Partnership was created to do which of the following?
   a. Protect institutions from lawsuits
   b. Advise hospitalized patients of their rights
   c. Prevent patients from making bad decisions
   d. Give autonomy to alternate decision makers
   e. Advise ambulatory patients of their rights

4. According to the Patient Care Partnership, what should patients expect when they are hospitalized?
   a. High-quality care.
   b. Protection of privacy.
   c. A clean and safe environment.
   d. All of the above.
   e. None of the above.

5. Which of the following actions violate patient confidentiality?
   a. Discussing a patient case in a public elevator
   b. Disclosing the results of diagnostic tests to friends of the patient
   c. Allowing public access to electronically stored patient information
   d. All of the above
   e. a and c above

6. What is wrong with a research review board composed of four male physicians?
   a. A board must have at least five members.
   b. More than one type of profession must be represented.
   c. Both men and women must be members.
   d. All of the above.
   e. None of the above.

7. The primary purpose of an institutional review board is to do which of the following?
   a. Judge the scientific merit of proposed research
   b. Locate funding sources for proposed research
   c. Safeguard the rights and welfare of human subjects
   d. Analyze the results of studies
   e. Protect the rights of researchers

8. Which one of the following is an optional element of informed consent?
   a. Additional costs to the subject for participating in the study
   b. An estimate of the expected duration of the subject's participation in the study
   c. Alternatives to participating in the study
   d. Whom to contact for answers to questions about the research subject's rights
   e. A statement that participation in the study is voluntary

9. Accepting gifts from pharmaceutical industry involves which of the following ethical principles?
   a. Justness
   b. Obligation
   c. Respect
   d. a and b above
   e. None of the above

10. Which of the following statements regarding living wills is false?
   a. Living wills provide specific information regarding medical treatment the patient does or does not want to have at the end of life.
   b. Living wills often must be interpreted.
   c. Living wills appoint a proxy.
   d. Living wills may become outdated.
   e. Living wills provide patients with the means to influence future treatment decisions.

References

1. Tempkin O, Temkin CL: *Ancient medicine: selected papers of Ludwig Edelstein*, Baltimore, 1967, Johns Hopkins University.
2. Knoepfler JF: Eidesformein für Arzt, Apotheker Hebammen, Wundarzt und Frauenwirt zu Amberg, *Arch Gesch Med* 11:318, 1919.
3. A code of ethics adopted by the Philadelphia College of Pharmacy, *Am J Pharm* 20:148-151, 1848.
4. *Code of ethics for pharmacists*, Washington, DC, 1995, American Pharmaceutical Association.
5. Vottero LD: The code of ethics for pharmacists, *Am J Health-Syst Pharm* 21:2096, 1995.
6. *Oath of a pharmacist*, Alexandria, VA, 1995, American Association of Colleges of Pharmacy.
7. King LS: IX. The AMA gets a new code of ethics, *JAMA* 249:1338-1342, 1983.
8. Principles of Medical Ethics. Available at: www.ama-asn.org/ama/pub/category. Accessed August 8, 2002.
9. Kelly C: *Dimensions of professional nursing*, New York, 1962, Macmillan.
10. Codes of Ethics for Nurses. Available at: www.nursingworld.org/ethics/code. Accessed August 8, 2002.
11. *The Patient Care Partnership: understanding expectations, rights, and responsibilities*, Chicago, 2003, American Hospital Association.
12. Rothman DJ: Ethics and human experimentation, *N Engl J Med* 317:1195-1199, 1987.
13. *Trials of war criminals before the Nuremberg military tribunals under control council law* 10:181-182, October 1946-April 1949.
14. Committee on Medical Ethics, World Medical Association: Declaration of Helsinki. As amended by the 52nd General Assembly, Edinburgh, Scotland, October, 2000. The WMA General Assembly added a Note of Clarification on paragraph 29, Washington, 2002.
15. Code of Federal Regulations (Title 21, Volume 1). Revised as of April 1, 2002. Available at: www.fda.gov. Accessed August 8, 2002.
16. Herman SS: A noninstitutional review board comes of age, *IRB* 11:1-6, 1989.

17. Zoloth AM: The need for ethical guidelines for relationships between pharmacists and the pharmaceutical industry, *Am J Hosp Pharm* 48:551-552, 1991.
18. Goldfinger SE: Physicians and the pharmaceutical industry, *Ann Intern Med* 112:624-626, 1990.
19. Chren M-M, Landefeld S, Murray TH: Doctors, drug companies, and gifts, *JAMA* 262:3448-3451, 1989.
20. ASHP guidelines on pharmacists' relationships with industry, *Am J Hosp Pharm* 49:154, 1992.
21. PhRMA Code on Interactions with Healthcare Professionals. Available at: www.phrma.org. Accessed November 14, 2002.
22. *Consolidated omnibus budget reconciliation act of* 1990, Pub. Law No. 101-508, Paragraphs 4206, 4751.
23. Danis M et al: A prospective study of advance directives for life-sustaining care, *N Engl J Med* 324:882-888, 1991.
24. Annas GJ: The health care proxy and the living will, *N Engl J Med* 324:1210-1213, 1991.
25. Smedira NG et al: Withholding and withdrawal of life support from the critically ill, *N Engl J Med* 322:309-315, 1990.

Answer Key for Self-Assessment Questions APPENDIX

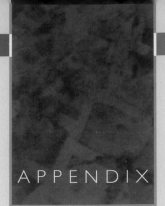

Chapter 1

1. e
2. d
3. b
4. a
5. d
6. c
7. c
8. b
9. d
10. d

Chapter 2

1. d
2. b
3. d
4. e
5. a
6. c
7. c
8. e
9. a
10. d

Chapter 3

1. c
2. d
3. e
4. d
5. b
6. d
7. a
8. d
9. a
10. b

Chapter 4

1. c
2. c
3. d
4. b
5. d
6. e
7. a
8. c
9. c
10. b

Chapter 5

1. d
2. b
3. a
4. c
5. e
6. b
7. a
8. c
9. d
10. e

Chapter 6

1. b
2. a
3. d
4. b
5. d
6. c
7. b
8. a
9. d
10. a

Chapter 7
1. e
2. c
3. d
4. c
5. b
6. a
7. a
8. c
9. e
10. a

Chapter 8
1. e
2. c
3. b
4. c
5. a
6. d
7. a
8. c
9. b
10. d

Chapter 9
1. d
2. a
3. d
4. a
5. b
6. c
7. d
8. d
9. c
10. d

Chapter 10
1. a
2. e
3. b
4. d
5. d
6. d
7. c
8. a
9. d
10. c

Index

Page numbers followed by f indicate figures;
t, tables; b, boxes.